Ethics by Committee

Ethics by Committee

A Textbook on Consultation, Organization, and Education for Hospital Ethics Committees

Edited by
D. Micah Hester

ROWMAN & LITTLEFIELD PUBLISHERS, INC.
Lanham • Boulder • New York • Toronto • Plymouth, UK

ROWMAN & LITTLEFIELD PUBLISHERS, INC.

Published in the United States of America
by Rowman & Littlefield Publishers, Inc.
A wholly owned subsidary of The Rowman & Littlefield Publishing Group, Inc.
4501 Forbes Boulevard, Suite 200, Lanham, Maryland 20706
www.rowmanlittlefield.com

Estover Road, Plymouth PL6 7PY, United Kingdom

British Library Cataloguing in Publication Information Available

Library of Congress Cataloging-in-Publication Data

Ethics by committee : a textbook on consultation, organization, and education for
    hospital ethics committees / edited by D. Micah Hester.
      p. ; cm.
    Includes bibliographical references and index.
    ISBN-13: 978-0-7425-5045-2 (cloth : alk. paper)
    ISBN-10: 0-7425-5045-1 (cloth : alk. paper)
    ISBN-13: 978-0-7425-5046-9 (pbk. : alk. paper)
    ISBN-10: 0-7425-5046-X (pbk. : alk. paper)
    1. Medical ethics committees 2. Hospitals—Moral and ethical aspects.
  3. Hospital care—Moral and ethical aspects. 4. Medical ethics. I. Hester, D.
  Micah. [DNLM: 1. Ethics Committees, Clinical. 2. Hospitals—ethics. 3. Ethics,
  Institutional. WX 150 E839 2008]
    R725.3.E89 2008
    174.2—dc22

                                                        2007020163

Printed in the United States of America

∞™ The paper used in this publication meets the minimum requirements of
American National Standard for Information Sciences—Permanence of Paper
for Printed Library Materials, ANSI/NISO Z39.48-1992.

Contents

Preface

If you are perusing this book, chances are that you are considering becoming a member of a hospital ethics committee (HEC),[1] are already a member of an HEC, or have been asked to help educate an HEC. If you are considering membership in an HEC, you probably are wondering (a) what is an HEC really, (b) how does it function, (c) what do I need to know to participate, and finally (d) why should I participate? The chapters in this book are developed to help answer (a) through (c), but indirectly you may also discover an answer for (d) as well. If, however, you are already a member of an HEC, you may be asking what you have gotten yourself into or how might you better prepare yourself for whatever you have gotten yourself into. Again, this book is intended to help. Finally, if you are asked to help educate an HEC, well, the purpose of this book should be obvious . . . I hope.

HEC members are a diverse group of individuals. They perform different professional tasks within the institution (physician, nurse, administrator, chaplain, social worker, risk management, and so forth), and even outside the institution (lay-community members, outside legal counsel, even academic philosophers). Each person comes with a wealth and variety of experiences, and this provides for a breadth of perspectives for the committee, and yet it is this diversity of backgrounds that also requires HEC members to educate themselves as ethics committee members. Most members, while they know well their own profession, have rarely studied in depth ethical theory or even the narrower field of medical ethics. However, no matter your interest level or experience in ethics, understanding how hospitals and medical care raise unique ethical concerns can be of help.

Ethics, it should be noted, is not simply learned experientially; it is not simply handed down as maxims and clichés from elders or experts. It is not as easy as following standards of practice or being a good person. It is a body of considered concepts that have gone through years of careful consideration. And yet, these concepts alone settle nothing by themselves; all ethical quandaries require not just the consideration of ethical concepts but also the use of deliberative methods to think through the unique features presented by medicine and professional conduct with each case, policy, and issue.

The chapters that follow are intended to provide educationally useful and relevant material for the wide spectrum of HEC members as they address the typical three charges of an HEC: consultation, education, and policy review/development—though not every HEC is so charged. The sections of the book reflect these three responsibilities, though the number of chapters is decidedly weighted to consultation and clinical issues, as these aspects of HEC practice tend to cause the most stress and concern for HEC members—even though the majority of time and effort of HECs is rarely used for consultation.

Further, each chapter of this book is authored by different individuals. Like the membership of HECs they try to help, the chapters demonstrate a variety of perspectives not in order to confuse or debate but to broaden and elucidate otherwise complex issues for HEC members (a clear example of this is the chapters by Shelton/Bjarnadottir and Finder/Bliton). Specifically, the authors have been chosen not because their perspectives agree with the editor or with each other but because the authors have demonstrated in their previous work the ability to educate effectively concerning the difficult and complex ethics issues that face HECs. Each chapter is designed to stand alone, offering upfront key points and concluding with questions for further reflection. The key points should help focus individual study, while the questions can be used to provoke group discussions of the issues raised relative to particular institutional experience and environment. Further, where appropriate, cross-reference to other chapters is provided.

It is hoped that the design of the book will make it easy to use the text as part of a regular process of education by and for an HEC (a chapter per month for the committee will complete the task in a little over one year), and it is intended that the chapters be taken not only as insightful in themselves but also as stimulants for discussion within the committee itself.

⎯⎯∞⎯⎯

This project began because I grew concerned for new members of HECs, since some are asked within weeks of joining the committee to participate in covering the committee pager for HEC consults. Many committees have only minimal educational material—for example, a couple of articles culled by a previous chair. Of course, not all HECs are so designed, and several have robust educational material and curricula. Unfortunately, far too many do not have the resources to develop good education for their members.

It is surprising that the ubiquity of HECs in hospitals has not resulted in more material specifically targeted to HEC education. By no means should this comment be taken to imply that no good material is available; there is. However, it is typically hard to find, only rarely is targeted in a specific way to HEC members, or is very new to the market. This book is consciously developed in light of the needs and experiences of HECs.

In developing this text, as editor I have incurred many debts, several I will probably forget to repay here, but below is list of individuals I owe my gratitude.

First, I owe each of the chapter authors herein. I met with nothing but quick and positive interest even when those I asked to write could not fit it into their busy schedules. Those who have written chapters are no less busy, and I am grateful that they were able to prioritize this project, taking up the charge to keep the material educationally accessible. Clearly, this book is theirs and not mine, in the most important sense.

Second, others helped discuss with me what should be the content of the book, the organization of the table of contents, and the specific content of each chapter. Though I apologize should I forget someone, these people, not otherwise published as chapter authors, are: Mark Aulisio, Paul Ford, Whit Hall, Diane Hoffman, Karen Kovach, Steve Leuthner, Alex London, Robert Talisse, and Patricia Werhane as well as members of my own local HECs, specifically, Martha Chamness and Danna Carver at UAMS and Del Farris, Bonnie Kitchens, and Bonnie Taylor at ACH.

Third, I need to thank the institutions—UAMS and ACH—that employ me and make my work possible though financial and administrative support. And specifically, individuals who have been thoroughly involved with me at UAMS on this project are my boss, Chris Hackler, and our division administrative assistant, Carol VanPelt.

Fourth, I would be remiss if I did not thank Rowman & Littlefield for agreeing to publish this manuscript with only a table of contents, a proposal, and a promise. In particular, former philosophy acquisitions editor (and strong backer of bioethics publication), Eve DeVaro Fowler, was the initial champion of this project at R&L, and her efforts should be recognized not only by me but by all the readers of this text as she shepherded this project through the process of getting a contract, and it was getting a contract that made securing chapter authors possible. Even after changes at R&L, the publisher has continued to be supportive of this project, and I want to thank specifically Jon Sisk and Ross Miller in this regard.

Finally, I always wish to thank my family, Kelly, Emily, and Joshua, for their love and support.

D. Micah Hester, PhD
University of Arkansas for Medical Sciences
Arkansas Children's Hospital

NOTE

1. While some people, institutions, and texts use broader terms like "institutional ethics committee" or "healthcare ethics committee," throughout this book we have chosen to use the term "hospital ethics committee" or "HEC" to designate an institutional committee in any healthcare–providing institution whose task it is to consider ethical issues within the institution. This choice, while linguistically restrictive, recognizes that the vast majority of these committees are specifically hospital-based. However, ethics committees in nursing homes or other chronic care facilities, for example, should also find educationally useful material herein.

1

Introduction

What Should an HEC Look and Act Like?

Chris Hackler and D. Micah Hester

ETHICS IN THE HOSPITAL: HOW DID WE GET HERE?

A child lies in the neonatal intensive care unit of a local hospital, having been born twelve weeks premature. For three weeks, she has been on a ventilator, assessed by pulmonologists, cardiologists, neurologists, and other specialists. She has dedicated nursing care, and her neonatologist visits the bedside daily. Her doctors agree that there is no realistic hope she will survive intensive care. While avoiding absolute pronouncements, they try to explain to the parents that their daughter is not responding to the treatment she is receiving, that in all likelihood she will not leave the hospital alive, and that the treatment necessarily involves considerable discomfort and even pain. Her young and bewildered parents, holding fast to a faith that their child will recover, request that the staff continue all aggressive treatments. This is difficult for some of the nurses, who consider the care to be "medically futile" and simply prolonging her suffering. They ask their supervisor about the hospital policy on futile care and are told there is none. The doctors are confused by what "futility" would mean in this situation and are not sure if they are legally and ethically bound to provide what the parents demand. When they approach the parents about shifting to "comfort care," the parents become confused and angry that it might mean abandoning their child's only hope of survival. They insist that all aggressive measures continue.

The atmosphere surrounding this case is charged with emotion and frustration, intensified by confusion, ambiguity, wishful thinking, and conflicting duties. Perhaps it would benefit from a dispassionate review by a group that is familiar with cases like this. Such a group might diffuse tensions, clarify the meaning of terms like "medical futility" and "comfort care," and suggest a way to reconcile conflicting obligations. They might then create educational programs to prepare the staff for similar situations in the future. They might even develop policies that would help resolve future conflicts that appear intractable. These three activities in fact constitute the typical charge of a hospital ethics committee (HEC).

The idea of an institutional *committee* to address ethical problems is a relatively recent one. Of course there is a long tradition of thinking about the ethical dimensions of the health care professions, dating at least to the famous oath of Hippocrates around the fourth century B.C.E. Young physicians since then have pledged to strive above all to benefit their patients and to refrain from any harm or injustice to the patient or family. This core commitment to the individual patient's welfare served as an ethical compass throughout ancient and medieval times. It seemed sufficient until about the middle of the previous century, when a number of important developments in both medical research and medical treatment shook the world of health care ethics and stimulated vigorous reflection about the very foundations of biomedical ethics.

Medical Research

At midcentury the world learned about unconscionable experiments conducted on captive populations against their will by German and Japanese doctors in the name of medical science. Two decades later the problem resurfaced within the scientific community with the publication of an article describing a number of apparently unethical experiments that had been conducted in the United States and published in leading medical journals (Beecher 1966). Then in 1972, the public learned that a study of untreated syphilis had been conducted for four decades on a group of unwitting black males in rural Alabama by the U.S. Public Health Service, with the cooperation of doctors from the medical school at the Tuskegee Institute. It seemed clear that the subjects did not understand the purpose of the study, that they thought they were receiving care for their illness when they were not, and that little was done to dispel that misunderstanding.[1]

Responding to intense publicity surrounding disclosure of the Tuskegee Study, as it came to be known, Congress established the National Commission for the Protection of Human Subjects of Biomedical and Behavioral Research (the Research Commission) with a threefold mission: formulate the basic ethical principles that should guide research with human subjects, study specific areas of ethical controversy, and recommend some practical steps to protect the rights of research subjects. The commission found three basic principles that should govern research with human subjects (respect for persons, beneficence, and justice); issued reports on such topics as research with children and fetuses; and, in response to the third charge, endorsed a system of peer review of research. The concept of peer review had been developing during the late 1960s in federal agencies such as the Public Health Service and the National Institutes of Health, later joined by the Department of Health and Human Services (DHHS) and the Food and Drug Administration (FDA). The Research Commission recommended combining these initiatives into one common federal system, which was done by DHHS and FDA in 1981 through the so-called Common Rule. The new system requires approval by an Institutional Review Board (IRB) before research with human subjects can be initiated. The IRB must examine each research proposal to gauge conformity to ethical principles and, through continuing review, to assure itself that the rights of research participants are respected for the duration of the research study. In addition to research experts, IRBs must have members who are neither research scientists nor institutional employees. This concept of an institutional ethics review committee was later applied, with significant modification, to the clinical setting.

Medical Treatment

Medical practice changed dramatically during the last half of the previous century, as new technologies gave rise to new ethical dilemmas. Organ transplantation, especially the possibility of heart transplantation, created the need to reconsider the traditional definition of death, which was based on the irreversible cessation of cardiac function. New life-prolonging technologies emerged, such as kidney dialysis, that were both scarce and expensive, creating disturbing choices about who would live and who would die. The new mechanical ventilators could support biological life well beyond the permanent loss of consciousness. New technologies continued to emerge that could further postpone the moment of death. The public sensed a loss of control over technology that was expressed not only in religious and philosophical terms, but in drama, fiction, and the visual arts. The moment of death was increasingly seen as a matter of human choice for which we seemed ill prepared. In 1978 Congress responded to the public's disquiet by creating the President's Commission for the Study of Ethical Problems in Medicine and Biomedical and Behavioral Research (President's Commission).

Although the Research Commission and the President's Commission were established to address different areas of concern, there is a notable similarity in their results. The President's Commission began by articulating the basic concepts and values that would guide its work, its three principles clearly resonating with those of the Research Commission.[2] The President's Commission issued a number of influential reports as well on such topics as defining death, forgoing life-sustaining treatment, and making healthcare decisions generally. Finally, much as the Research Commission recommended a system of peer review committees to safeguard the welfare and rights of subjects of biomedical research, the President's Commission suggested that hospitals establish interdisciplinary committees to provide guidance in difficult treatment decisions, especially those at the end of life.

While the President's Commission did not recommend the immediate formation of an ethics committee in every hospital, it did support the establishment of interdisciplinary committees to help educate hospital personnel about ethical issues, formulate hospital policies or guidelines, and review or help make decisions about the care of individual patients (DFLST 160–70). In making its recommendation, the President's Commission cited earlier experiences with similar committees. It mentioned the involvement of community representatives in Seattle to help select among candidates for dialysis, literally making life-or-death decisions in the days before dialysis became widely available. It also endorsed the approach the New Jersey Supreme Court took to decision making for incapacitated patients in the *Quinlan* case, leaving the decision to the patient's guardians in consultation with the "ethics committee" it seemed to assume most hospitals had (DFLST, 155–156).[3] It is important to stress at the outset, however, that the functions of research ethics committees and clinical ethics committees have differed in one critical respect: research committees make decisions whether or not research may proceed, whereas the traditional mandate of clinical ethics committees is only to educate, facilitate, mediate, and perhaps advise about particular cases. Clinical decisions remain in the hands of physicians, patients, and families.

The Idea Takes Hold

A number of influential organizations have subsequently endorsed the concept of HECs, including the American Hospital Association (1986) and the American Medical Association (Ethical and Judicial Council 1985). But the most influential proponent has been the Joint Commission on the Accreditation of Healthcare Organizations (Joint Commission, or JCAHO), which began in 1992 to require some kind of formal structure (in their words, "a mechanism") to assure that ethical issues in patient care were addressed in an effective fashion. The Joint Commission did not mandate a committee but did mention an HEC as one obvious way to fulfill the requirement. The result was a rapid increase in the number of HECs in hospitals of all sizes. At the turn of the new century most hospitals had an ethics committee at least in name. Given the variation in size, mission, geographic location, and financial stability, one might suppose that the committees would vary widely in size, function, energy, and effectiveness. That supposition would be entirely correct.

Exact numbers are not available, but a conservative estimate would be that 30,000 people (and probably double that) in the United States currently serve in some manner on an HEC (Fox et al. 2007). Since there are only around 1,600 members of the American Society for Bioethics and Humanities, the dominant professional organization in bioethics, it is apparent that the great majority of HEC members would not identify themselves as professionals in the field of healthcare ethics and thus may find themselves uncomfortable in their role as a "go-to" person for ethical concerns in the hospital. The present volume hopes to reduce that discomfort by clarifying the roles of HEC members, suggesting ways to prepare for those roles, and addressing some of the organizational issues that ethics committees face.

WHAT DOES AN HEC DO?

The traditional threefold mission of an HEC has not changed substantially since the President's Commission formulated it in 1983. The most visible and controversial role is to consult on difficult clinical decisions. Equally important, though sometimes forgotten, are the other two functions: formulating institutional policies to guide the professional staff in making ethical decisions, and educating hospital personnel about these policies and about healthcare ethics in general. For example, the case at the beginning alluded to all three functions: the HEC might be called in to consult with the staff and parents, it might be asked to develop a policy for conflict resolution, and it might be asked to provide staff with further education about the ethical and legal considerations. We will discuss the three roles in reverse order.

Education

As we have seen, the great majority of HEC members probably have little academic training or other formal background in the field of healthcare ethics. Yet their position on the HEC implies that they are prepared to help others resolve ethical problems. Thus they feel the need for some education to give them confidence in their ability to help, and to give them credibility in the eyes of their colleagues who might turn to them. For these reasons, the first task of an HEC is to provide education to its own members. There are several ways to do this, depending on the resources available to the committee. Academic medical centers can provide consultants to structure an education program. Conferences, seminars, and workshops are frequently aimed at HEC members. If at all possible, an HEC should have a small budget to finance its self-education. Handbooks, textbooks, and casebooks are also available that can provide content for a self-structured study group (of course, the book you are reading is specifically designed to do so). Some committees do not offer themselves for service until a period of self-education is finished, whereas others prefer to start to work while the educational activity is still underway. In either case, the committee should resist the view that its education is ever complete, as the field of healthcare ethics is vast and continues to expand. There are always new issues to confront or old issues with a novel twist. Even highly trained professionals in medical ethics are limited in their knowledge of specific issues and preparation for specific tasks. Some committees make time in their regular meetings for an educational component, devoting fifteen to thirty minutes to a discussion of a timely topic, policy, or case. If possible, a reading room with selected journals, texts, and casebooks in healthcare ethics should be available to committee members and everyone else in the hospital. But since no collection of readings can cover all problems, members should know how to conduct a computer search of the bioethics literature on a particular topic. (Readers will find more information on bioethics resources in the Further Resources section at the end of the book as well as in the Works Cited section of each chapter.)

An HEC should also provide education to the entire hospital community. When it feels prepared, it should advertise its availability through hospital publications and in department meetings, giving examples of the kinds of problems it might help to resolve. When a policy is adopted or revised that has ethical dimensions, the committee should offer to present the policy and discuss its rationale. If it has a budget or access to funding, the committee can invite outside speakers to address perennial issues in healthcare ethics like surrogate decision making or the allocation of scarce resources. Such initiatives can forestall problems that arise from lack of awareness and can enhance the visibility and credibility of the committee. In designing such programs, the HEC should be mindful of all professionals in the hospital, such as social workers and allied health providers, who are sometimes overlooked. (See chapter 10 for more on the responsibility of committee education.)

Policy Review

Every hospital has policies that deal with ethical concerns. Some are obviously ethical in nature, such as policies that govern advance directives, orders not to attempt resuscitation, and identification of appropriate surrogates. Others that are not overtly ethical in content may still have ethical dimensions—for example, policies concerning admission, discharge, and transfer of patients. An HEC should be careful in determining which policies to review and how it conducts its review. In general, ethics committees can take the lead with policies that affect all or most clinical departments in the institution—policies dealing with informed consent, advance directives, and surrogate decision making, for example. But the committee should be careful to work with other departments that will be especially affected by a given policy. It would be inappropriate, for example, to write a policy on resuscitation without involving pulmonary specialists, cardiologists, and other intensivists. Care should be taken in reviewing a policy that originated in a particular unit of the organization. Feathers can be ruffled if another unit's policy is reviewed without a specific invitation or charge.

Ethics committees do some of their most important work in formulating and reviewing hospital policies. The ethical climate of any institution is determined in large part by the policies it adopts (assuming that its practices are congruent with its policies). Moreover, by offering reasonably clear guidelines for difficult situations, good policies help individuals make good decisions and thus prevent some ethical problems from arising. In fact many ethical problems can be prevented if individuals are informed about ethical precepts and have sound policies to guide them. Since it is usually better to avoid problems than to have to solve them, we should never overlook the two "preventive ethics" functions of education and policy review. Although they involve hard, behind-the-scenes work and may not have all of the cachet of case consultation, they should be included explicitly as equal aspects of the charge of any hospital ethics committee. In many ways, education and policy review are like public health and preventive medicine, which are less glamorous than acute care medicine but contribute more to the overall health of a society. (For more on policy, see chapter 13.)

No matter how much preventive medicine or ethics we have done, however, when an acute problem arises, we need individuals with special education and experience to help deal with it. For an ethics committee, this means case consultation.

Case Consultation

Although JCAHO requires a mechanism for addressing ethical issues that arise in the hospital, it does not specifically require an ethics committee. The function of education could be facilitated by an ethics education specialist, for example, and policy review could be conducted by an ethics officer in the administration. Similarly, ethics consultation could be conducted by an ethics consultant. This approach has in fact been used successfully by a number of hospitals, typically large institutions with the resources to support specialists and support staff in this area. One advantage of the "ethics consultant approach" is that it brings the expertise and experience of a specialist to the task. An ideal ethics consultant would be an individual who has studied healthcare ethics, has demonstrated competence in an academic discipline that informs the field, such as philosophy or religion, and is familiar with the clinical setting. Another advantage is that the consultant can respond quickly to a request for help and can meet with key individuals in an efficient manner, on their own turf according to their various schedules. As a specialist of sorts, the ethics consultant may enjoy a more immediate acceptance by his or her colleagues in health care. Physicians especially are familiar with the concept of expert consultants and might more readily acknowledge the legitimacy of an ethics consultant as opposed to a hospital committee.

A more common approach, however, especially in small- to medium-size hospitals, is to have a multidisciplinary committee that conducts all three activities, with consultations conducted by the whole committee. The volume of requests for consultation is usually small in the early years of an HEC and would not support a specialized consultation service. There is nothing inherently wrong with the "whole committee" approach, and it still serves many established committees well. It ensures a variety of ethical and professional perspectives, and it gathers partial expertise from a larger number of individuals with limited study of healthcare ethics. If they feel the need, committees may initiate informal arrangements with specialists from nearby academic health centers to assist their deliberations as needed. A drawback of the whole committee model, however, is that it can be cumbersome. When the committee is conducting a consultation, everyone must come to the committee to be heard. It is quite a challenge to get a committee of busy professionals together with the patient's doctors, nurses, and social workers in a timely manner. Moreover, it can be a daunting experience for patients or their families to enter a room filled with white coats and start answering questions, no matter how benign and concerned the committee wants to appear!

As an HEC grows in experience and size, it may want to consider a third approach to ethics consultation: a smaller group that is constituted by the HEC specifically to serve its consultative function. Members of the group are chosen for their special abilities and ready availability to provide help. This "team model" attempts to incorporate some of the best features of both the individual consultant and the whole committee models. Like the individual consultant, a small group that is "on call" is able to respond quickly to an urgent need, can be flexible in meeting with involved parties in various locations in the hospital, and is less intimidating to patients and families. Larger groups such as the whole HEC are generally more cumbersome in this regard. Members of the group would be chosen for their availability, of course, but primarily for their experience and the particular skills they would bring to the team. As an interdisciplinary group, it would be expected to contain different ethical perspectives as well as differing sets of skills and experience. It is possible that the team would provide a more comprehensive package of knowledge, skill, and experience than an individual consultant would provide.

The consult group may be constituted in different ways. It may be composed only of members of the HEC, or it might include individuals chosen for a particular skill that would be valuable in this setting, such as a psychiatrist who is experienced in assessing decisional capacity or in mediating disputes. However it is constituted, the consult group should be responsible to the parent HEC, reporting on its activities at regular intervals. (For more on consult-group issues, see Smith et al. 2004.)

No matter which model of consultation is adopted, the consult group should give thought to the goal of its consultations. Three outcomes are commonly sought: clarification, conflict resolution, and treatment recommendation. The first goal is always appropriate. Ethical dilemmas can be complex and emotionally charged, making it difficult for those immediately involved to think clearly about them. A careful analysis of the conflicting beliefs, values, and commitments that give rise to a dilemma is the first step toward resolving it. It can be helpful to develop some kind of method or framework for achieving analytical clarity, perhaps a checklist of steps to take and points to consider as one gathers and processes information about the case. (An example of a consultation method is presented in chapter 4 by Shelton and Bjarnadottir, who extend and adapt the "four boxes" model developed by Jonsen, Siegler, and Winslade [2002].) A certain base of knowledge about ethical concepts and landmark legal cases is also necessary if consultation is to be credible and effective. The *Core Competencies* document published by the American Society for

Bioethics and Humanities (1998) provides a convenient summary of the knowledge and skills that are critical to this important goal of case consultation.

Sometimes analysis and clarification are all that are needed, especially if the problem is lack of knowledge, clarity, or confidence in one's decision. At other times, however, there is a more deep-seated disagreement based on conflicting concerns that cannot be resolved by clarification. Some committees then take a more active role in mediating the dispute, trying to facilitate a mutually acceptable resolution to the conflict. Conflict resolution through mediation is always an appropriate goal for an HEC, and every consultation group should be prepared to attempt it. Successful mediation can honor the autonomy and preserve the dignity of all parties while demonstrating the utility of the consult service, producing a "win-win-win" outcome. The mediation aspect of case consultation is discussed in greater detail by Dubler and Liebman (2004).

The third possible role for a consult service is to make a treatment recommendation. As indicated earlier, HECs do not make treatment decisions unless they have been delegated explicit authority to do so. When would a consult service venture beyond the relatively safe realms of clarification and mediation? There are at least three kinds of situations that may call for a more active stance. First and most obviously, the group may be asked for advice. When physicians ask for a medical consult, they are asking for an expert opinion, whether, for example, a given procedure would be medically justifiable. Similarly, a physician may ask the HEC for an opinion whether a given procedure would be ethically justifiable. It is also possible that a patient or family would come to the HEC with the same question. There is no inherent reason why an HEC should not attempt to answer such a question. Second, attempts at mediation of a conflict between physician and family may be unsuccessful. At this point a decision still needs to be made, informed, one would hope, by the best ethical reasoning available. If the consulting group has an opinion about the matter, it seems appropriate that they express it. Finally, and perhaps most controversially, the consulting group may feel that the outcome of their mediation efforts is not ethically supportable. The physician and family, for example, may agree to a course of treatment that seems to violate an important right or interest of the patient. While such outcomes are probably quite rare, they are certainly possible.

Having selected among the individual, committee, and team models of consultation and defined more or less the kinds of outcomes to be expected from consultation, an HEC needs to consider whether it will use a specified methodology in conducting case consultations. Should a common analytical framework be developed or adopted by the committee? The methodology an HEC employs may well emerge from the group's self-education phase. In any case, new members of the committee will need to be educated about whatever analytical framework the committee decides to adopt.

WHAT DOES AN HEC LOOK LIKE?

As noted, the Joint Commission makes no pronouncements about how to constitute a "mechanism" to address ethical concerns. Thus there are no authoritative guidelines about how the committee should be developed—its administrative location, its charge, and its membership. In looking at what benefits a committee might bring to its institution, however, the design of the committee begins to come clear.

Location and Accountability

One of the first decisions to be made about an ethics committee is: Whose committee is it? All institutional committees are established by a particular administrative unit. They are given a purpose or charge and are responsible for reporting on their activities to the parent unit. Most HECs have been created by the medical staff or the hospital administration, though some have been established by the hospital's board of directors. Although it may not be a crucial decision, the location of the HEC in the institution's administrative structure can have some practical consequences, since guidelines for constituting and operating the committee may vary according to the group to which it is responsible. In some hospitals, for example, medical staff committees must be chaired by physicians, thus restricting the options for filling this important position. On the other hand, as a medical staff committee intent on quality improvement, it may be easier to shield proceedings of the HEC from any potential legal scrutiny.

In some institutions, the organized medical staff is skeptical or even mistrustful of the concept of an ethics committee. In such cases, it might be advisable to establish the HEC as a unit of the hospital administration. If it is an administrative committee, however, its purpose must not be perceived as making the hospital run smoothly. The third possibility, board committee status, can carry both positive and negative messages. On the one hand, the HEC is answerable only to the highest authority, which gives it significant status. On the other, this may carry the implication that its purpose is to oversee and perhaps report on medical and administrative decisions, creating distance from the very people it wants to help. The foregoing are only sketchy ideas that indicate some of the concerns relevant to administrative placement of an HEC in the organization's structure. The best place for an HEC to be located may involve many subtle factors that vary from place to place and may change over time in any given institution.

Leadership

Committees are rarely effective if they do not have good leadership. Thus the chair of an HEC is always a critical position to fill. The chair will become the de facto face of the committee and should be someone who enjoys respect and credibility among all professions in the institution. The most important quality, however, is commitment to the idea of an HEC. The chair must believe in the mission of the committee and consider the position an important part of his or her job. Meetings will be perfunctory and unproductive unless the chair takes care to construct a meaningful agenda. A certain esprit de corps is necessary for a committee to function well, a spirit that is engendered and nurtured by an energetic and committed chair (and regular meetings). The chair represents the committee and keeps it visible to the rest of the staff and administration. An unseen HEC will also be unused. When individuals contact the committee for help, it is the chair who must decide how to respond. An appropriate response builds confidence in the ability of the HEC to provide useful assistance.

Where should one look for a suitable chair? Other things being equal, it is probably better if the HEC is chaired by a physician, if one can be recruited who has the characteristics just described. A physician chair tends to have more immediate credibility with physician colleagues, perhaps making it easier for them to call on the committee for help. As we have seen, in some institutions, the committee is under the auspices of the medical staff, and only a physician is allowed to function as chair. However, in other hospitals, no such rules exist, and in those cases, even community members have been known to chair the committee. As with committee membership in general, there are no hard-and-fast rules; committee founders need to assess the available resources and the pragmatics of the institution to determine who should chair the HEC.

Membership

An ethics committee, as opposed to individual consultants and administrators or compliance officers, allows for an array of knowledge and perspectives to be brought to bear on consultation, education, and policy issues. Thus the committee should be multidisciplinary, composed of members with a variety of professional perspectives on clinical care (both physicians and nurses) and on broader social issues (for example, social workers and ethicists). Second, a committee allows for a variety of expertise. Since general familiarity with ethical issues in health care is clearly desirable, particular physicians and nurses with training or deep interest in ethical issues are obvious targets for membership. At the same time, policies or cases tend to cluster in or overly affect certain units. Thus, it might be important to have, say, a critical care specialist on the committee, as cases from the ICU are often fraught with ethical concern.

While special knowledge is desirable on the committee, three areas of expertise are controversial: law, religion, and business. Should a lawyer (or risk manager), chaplain, or administrator from the institution be named to the committee? In each of these cases, conflicts of interest are the primary concern. While ethics committees are *institutional* committees, they are charged to be "objective" in their deliberations, looking out for what is the best solution to a difficult case or complicated policy, not just what is best for the institution. Thus, some argue that the hospital administrator has too great a stake in the well-being of the institution to be sufficiently objective. Likewise, the job of the risk manager or hospital lawyer is to protect the legal interests of the institution and its employees. While these interests are certainly important, they must not be the focus of the ethics committee, which should concern itself above all with the ethical values at stake.

Chaplain membership can be a sensitive matter as well. The specific religious and value system that a chaplain or local minister brings to the institution may not be broadly representative, and a dogmatic preacher can tie a committee in knots. On the other hand, most hospital chaplains are ecumenical in spirit and highly skilled at ethical reasoning. In any case, chaplains are frontline caregivers who quickly become involved in the ethical struggles of the patients to whom they are ministering. As such, they can be valuable members, or at least allies, of the committee. Membership on the committee may also broaden their knowledge and sophistication about ethical issues. Of course, their effectiveness can be limited by the fact that they may already be involved in most cases because of the role they perform and, in a sense, be a stakeholder in the case at hand.

There is no settled opinion in the HEC community as to whether any or all of these positions should be built into the ethics committee. The conundrum is real. A committee needs to be aware of legal parameters to avoid leading individuals they are trying to help into legal danger. It needs to be aware of the limits of institutional resources to avoid giving advice that is unrealistic and potentially unjust. It also needs to be aware of religious or cultural values that underlie a patient's otherwise incomprehensible decision to refuse treatment. But it must not place the interests of the institution foremost in its deliberations, as the lawyer or administrator may be inclined to do. It must consider religious and cultural values while not assuming they are true or forcing them on individuals who do not share them. It is an unfortunate fact that committees tend to defer to a lawyer's pronouncements about the law, an administrator's assessment of possibilities, and a clergyman's vision of what is appropriate. While these concerns are important, they are only parts of the whole story that the committee should consider. The best solution would be to find professionals in each of these fields who can help the committee broaden its knowledge and vision while not preempting its deliberations or constricting its options.

Another unique category of membership is that of the "community member." While not a requirement, many HECs, perhaps structuring themselves after the IRB model, employ community members—that is, persons not directly associated with the institution. The purpose of the role is to provide a kind of corrective should the institutional members of the committee become insulated from public perceptions or too interested in institutional protection. This is a daunting role to perform. Like the professionals just discussed, it may be difficult to identify persons to fill the role. In fact, the person filling the role often has some relationship with the institution (ex-patient, former employee, spouse of an employee), raising questions whether that individual can adequately fulfill the intended role of the community member. Probably the only advice for *all* of these controversial positions is to consider the matter carefully in light of available local resources and periodically revisit the issue.

In addition to knowledge and position in the institution, a number of personal qualities are critical to the success of an HEC. Members must believe in the importance of the committee's work and be willing to devote significant time and energy to it. They should also try to take advantage of opportunities for self-education. Moreover, for an HEC to function smoothly and effectively, members must respect one another and the various perspectives they represent. A certain egalitarianism should pervade the committee's work. Differences of status within the organization should be left at the committee room door. It is cogency of reasoning that should matter, not position in the institution. Members should be respectful but not deferential to one another, and anyone who expects deference should be dropped from the committee.

Bylaws

Like any other working committee, an HEC needs a set of bylaws or a detailed committee charge to give it structure and allow for necessary changes in an orderly manner. In addition to leadership and categories of membership, the bylaws should address term of membership, frequency of meetings, and the scope of the three roles of education, policy review, and consultation.

Length of service on the committee can be an important matter. Short terms and a rapidly rotating membership will result in instability and inexperience, whereas indefinite or permanent membership may burden a committee with uninterested and unproductive members. The best solution is probably a compromise, such as fixed terms of two or three years with the possibility of reappointment. Uninvolved members can easily be dropped and committed ones retained as long as they contribute to the group.

Frequency of meetings is another item the bylaws should address. Regular meetings should be mandated. It is easy for overburdened professionals to slip into the "only when necessary" mode, which in effect means only when there is a consult to conduct. Without regular meetings, however, the "preventive" work of the committee—education and policy review—will be ignored. Self-education and self-assessment will also suffer, affecting the quality of the consults, and the committee will lose a sense of its continuing importance to the life of the hospital. Quarterly meetings are the minimum to retain a sense of continuity, with more frequent meetings highly desirable.

The bylaws should define as clearly as possible the role that the HEC is to play in all three of its primary activities. The educational function will probably be left entirely to the committee, to design and implement programs that it can offer on its own or through departmental meetings (again, having a budget for this purpose is highly desirable). The bylaws might, however, specify a base level of ethics education that committee members should have (see chapter 10). With respect to policy review, the HEC will probably be charged not to make changes but to recommend them to the administration or to the medical board. In this it is similar to every other committee in the institution, as committees are generally created to make recommendations rather than final decisions about policy matters. If there are particular policies the committee is to "own" or review regularly, they should be specified in the bylaws.

The most important function to clarify in the committee's bylaws is case consultation, since there may be uncertainty as to what kind of outcome to expect. Although in general, committees are charged to make recommendations to others, some are in fact constituted to make binding decisions about particular cases. As we have seen, for example, the IRB can either approve or reject research proposals. There is general agreement, however, that *clinical* decisions should not be made by a committee but should remain in the hands of physicians and families. Nevertheless there is sometimes considerable apprehension about the ethics committee taking control of a case when called to consult. Committee bylaws should specify that the committee is advisory only and does not make decisions about patient care. Some committees build this into their name (for example, "Medical Ethics Advisory Committee") to make clear the limit to their authority. There may be a small subset of cases that the committee is given explicit authority to decide; if so, these should be spelled out carefully in the committee bylaws.

CONCLUSION

The Hospital Ethics Committee is now a fixture in American hospitals, yet, like any complex institution, it is still defining itself. The concept has been scrutinized in the scholarly and professional literature for some twenty years, including several books and countless articles focused on the consultative function of an HEC. There are ethics committee networks in several states and regions of the country. There is no lack of resources to aid an institution in organizing, educating, or revivifying a moribund committee. In the end, however, the general idea of an HEC must be adapted to the particular structure, mission, and size of the institution and, just as important, to its professional and community resources. This book can help by presenting current thinking about major issues to be considered, indicating resources for further information, and suggesting ways to tailor an HEC to fit local conditions.

NOTES

1. Much has been written about this lengthy research project. For a historical account see James H. Jones, *Bad Blood: The Tuskegee Syphilis Experiment*, rev. ed. (NY: Free Press, 1992), and for an anthology of recent scholarship, see Susan M. Reverby, *Tuskegee's Truths* (Chapel Hill: UNC Press, 2000).

2. The first principle the President's Commission recognized was well-being, promoting the overall best interests of everyone involved. The commission stressed that patient well-being should be the primary focus, but that the well-being of others, including family, caregivers, and the larger community, is also ethically relevant. The second principle was self-determination or autonomy. Respecting this principle means giving patients information about their condition and about possible choices and honoring the choices that patients make. It also means safeguarding their privacy. The third principle is equity or justice, treating people fairly, or in an even-handed and nondiscriminatory manner.

3. We should note that the role the court assigned to the ethics committee was primarily to review the patient's prognosis, rather than clarify or help resolve the underlying ethical issue.

WORKS CITED

American Hospital Association. 1986. Guidelines: Hospital committees on biomedical ethics. In *Handbook for hospital ethics committees*, ed. J. W. Ross, 57, 110–11. Chicago, IL: American Hospital Publishing.

American Society for Bioethics and Humanities. 1998. *Core competencies for bioethics consultation*. Glenview, IL: American Society for Bioethics and Humanities.

Beecher, Henry K. Ethics and clinical research. *New England Journal of Medicine* 274 (1966): 1354–60.

Dubler, N., and C. Liebman. 2004. *Bioethics mediation: A guide to shaping shared solutions*. New York: United Hospital Funds of New York.

Ethical and Judicial Council. 1985. Guidelines for ethics committees in health care institutions. *JAMA* 253:2698–99.

Fox E., et al. 2007. Ethics consultation in United States hospitals: A national survey. *American Journal of Bioethics* 7 (2): 13–25.

Joint Commission on Accreditation of Healthcare Organizations. 1992. *Accreditation manual for hospitals, 1993 edition*. Oakbrook Terrace, IL: Joint Commission on Accreditation of Healthcare Organizations.

Jonsen, A., M. Siegler, and Winslade. 2002. *Clinical ethics: A practical approach to ethical decisions in clinical medicine*. 5th ed. McGraw-Hill.

President's commission for the study of ethical problems in medicine and biomedical and behavioral research. 1983. *Deciding to forego life-sustaining treatment*.

Smith, M. L., et al. 2004. Criteria for determining appropriate method for an ethics consultation. *HEC Forum* 16 (2): 95–113.

2

The "What?" and "Why?" of Ethics

D. Micah Hester

THE MEANING OF "ETHICS"

It is worth taking a moment, up front, to mention the "what" and "why" of ethics in medicine. Ethics, itself, has multiple meanings, and depending on the meaning you carry with you, it may be confusing, even frustrating, to be asked to consider ethics *education* itself.

First, many of us carry with us the colloquial meaning that "ethics" concerns how each individual deals with "right" and "wrong," "good" and "bad." We talk about our personal ethics, and frankly most, if not all, of us believe we are good people who have "ethics." This sense of ethics is tied closely to *values* and *character*.

Second, we recognize that as members of a profession we might be governed by "ethics." This governing is often manifest in "codes," but it also resides in our sense of what being a professional is all about—the responsibilities and obligations that come along with the actions we perform in our roles as healthcare professionals. This sense of ethics is often associated with judgments of what is *right* and *wrong*.

Third, we carry with us our values and interests, and we begin to recognize that others, too, have their own interests as well. Further, the roles we play, not only as professionals but as family members, friends, citizens, and religious (or nonreligious) believers, each carry corresponding obligations. Often, between personal interests, cultural values, and professional and relational obligations, it is not uncommon to find ourselves in conflict with others, with institutions, even with the many aspects of ourselves. Here conflicting concerns often lead to questions concerning ends we really should pursue and what means are appropriate in those pursuits. This sense of ethics can be characterized as weighing *good* and *bad*, *better* and *worse*.

No one of these three senses should be ignored or dominant. It is worth noting that each of us is a "values carrier" whether as a product of biology, nurturing, education, or some other means. Further, we do, in fact, find ourselves in relation to others—familial, professional, and so forth—and those relationships commit us to others and to expectations for which we are held accountable. Finally, in a finite universe of limited abilities and resources, with a plurality of individual and communal interests, we are confronted often by concerns for what we should do, and why.

Ethics, then, as addressed in this book, concerns each of these aspects of moral living—values (character), duties (roles), and goods (ends).

IS ETHICS EDUCATION USEFUL?

But now, you might ask yourself, "Why should I take the time to look at this? First, I have good values—I'm on an ethics committee, after all; I care. Second, medical professions do, in fact, have codes of ethics, and thus, there are already guidelines of ethically acceptable practice. Finally, is there really such a thing as developing an expertise in resolving ethical conflict?"

Each point captures an aspect of truth. Most of us do make ethically acceptable choices based on values grounded on morally worthy sources. Further, the profession of medicine has long concerned itself with ethical practice. And frankly, resolving ethical conflict is not always an easy task. Of course, it is this last claim that makes ethical reflection all the more important, but ethical reflection is incapable of stopping at the "borders" of the particular conflict in front of us. Each consideration raises issues of "principle" not just expediency, and thus, reconsideration of our professional obligations; and further, our individual values are implicated in our ethical decision making. Furthermore, it is also the case that our values and professional obligations are the products of past experiences, and thus, on the one hand, they are incapable of guaranteeing their clear applicability to any new situation and, on the other hand, are generalized to such an extent that what "applicability" even means comes into question.

For example, let us consider you to be a "good person," raised "well" with "good" values. Further, let us recognize that as a medical professional, you are under an obligation to act in the best interest of patients, and as a citizen, you are told that you should not kill another person. One day, a sixty-five-year-old oncology patient who has failed her third round of chemotherapy asks for your help in hastening her death. She states clearly to you that she finds her life insufferable, and that dying quickly while she still has some dignity is of utmost importance to her. Just relying on the fact that you are a "good" person and that you recognize professional obligations, how do these facts settle the moral issue for you? Frankly, they cannot. Now, this is not to say that they do not help you in determining the best thing to do, but these facts alone do not get you far enough. Even if your values and interests lean you toward helping her, you are stuck trying to determine whether doing so is best, and even if your responsibilities to the state bar you from assisting in someone's suicide, this does not tell you what forms of aid are acceptable, nor does the law settle the ethical tensions themselves—especially when the person who is suffering is also willing to die.

The point is that as ethically equipped as human beings are, it is problematic to think that education would not be helpful. No one of us has a hold on the whole of moral truth, and at the same time, each of us probably has some hold on an aspect of that truth. Ethics education, like all education, aims at developing habits of intelligent action to adjudicate both the amount of *and* lack of moral insight we have—recognizing that our own values have no better a priori claim to morality than the next person's. More importantly, given that everyone's character and the practices of every profession are subject to continual (if not cataclysmic) change requires a certain continual vigilance with respect to reflecting on whom we want to become, what we are willing to do, and how we should interact with those around us. Dedicated educational time can be especially useful in this endeavor as it affords participants opportunities to reflect without the pressures of pressing clinical needs and stresses. In short, dedicated education provides the space for intelligence to focus specifically on habits of ethical reflection, deliberation, and determination.

ETHICAL REFLECTION

While there are many ethical theories and methods that have been developed—Aristotle's virtue ethics, Kant's deontology, Mill's utilitarianism, Gilligan's ethics of care, principlism, casuistry, narrative ethics, and so forth, short of a full-blown course in ethical theory and method, no one would expect you to have a firm handle on these. However, this does not mean that theory and method are, therefore, unimportant. As mentioned earlier, none of our actions are performed in isolation, nor are policies written in a vacuum. Reasons and justifications are necessary components of ethical determinations, whether concerning particular situations or institutional policies. Further, consistency of considerations is not unimportant either. Consistent reasoning stems from justified principled positions, and those arise from long processes of inquiry into the moral life itself. It is not good enough simply to care about the consequences of our actions for some issues and about our dutiful obligations toward others on a whim. We must be able to account for the legitimacy of our use of methods and theories that underlie the deliberations we perform and decisions we make.

Closer to home, we might also say (along with members of the Columbia University philosophy department of the 1920s) that there is a "kind of progress possible through reflection in ethics" (Buermeyer et al. 1923, 323) which may be noted in four types: First, ethical reflection can bring our own values to light, "values which we might otherwise overlook" (323). Second, reflection aids in clarifying our aims and desires. Third, ethical reflection allows us to separate wheat from chaff, helping "us see what problems really are most vital, and thus bring[ing] us nearer to actual solutions" (324). And finally, fourth, reflection leads us to own our actions, making "our conduct more fully our own, more voluntary and less of a blind obedience to custom" (324).

While this book contains several chapters with more in-depth discussions about ethical reasoning (chapter 3) and practical methods (chapter 4), let me sketch out what I take to be the basic aspects of ethical reflection—those aspects that most clearly lead to the four types of progress noted above. This sketch is quite general, and thus, one virtue is that it should not conflict with the more detailed discussions that other authors provide herein. Further, it is purposefully developed to dovetail nicely with the way we think about most any medical issue, not just those that demand ethical reflection. What is presented, then, is the "scientific" method as it applies to ethical considerations, and such a broad reflective framework can help in ethical analysis, even when employing more specific methods.

1. **Confrontation with a problem (What issues are raised by the case?)**: When you hear about a case, what bothers you or strikes you as problematic? What values are being expressed? What principles are in tension? Where, how, and why does conflict occur?
2. **Define the problem (What is the central question of the case?)**: What is (are) the *central ethical question(s)* (CEQ) put by the case? While it may be necessary to address a fair number of questions in an ethical analysis of a case, a central ethical question is a *primary* ethical concern that *must* be addressed and answered if the physician is to know how to proceed. It should arise directly from the ethical tensions/problems that the individuals and context of this case pose. There can be *more than one* central question.
3. **Pose alternative responses to the problem (What answers are reasonable? What *claims* can be presented as answers?)**: What are the available (i.e., all possible, reasonable) answers to the central question(s)? That is, what might someone reasonably state as a legitimate solution to the ethical dilemmas posed by #2?
4. **Reason through the alternatives (What is the best answer and why?)**:
   a. *First step*: What are the best arguments supporting *each* of the answers you give in #3? What *support/warrant/backing* is there for each of the *claims* made in #3?
   b. *Second step*: Where are the arguments you describe weak or vulnerable to serious objection? What *qualifiers/exceptions* exist that weaken the *support* for each *claim*? Can they be strengthened to avoid objection, and if so, how?
   c. *Third step*: Given your work addressing #4a and #4b, which answer(s) to the central question(s) is (are) *best*? *Why*?
5. **Test/Implement the proposed solution (How should you execute your solution? What *qualifiers/exceptions* must be considered?)**: How should your chosen answer (#4c) to the central question be implemented given the *specifics of the case at hand*?

Are there practical/procedural concerns that must be addressed in order to employ what you have determined is the most ethical solution to the dilemma?

It is important to note that these five "aspects" of reflection are listed consecutively primarily for educational purpose—that is, in order to help in developing good habits of inquiry (see Dewey 1910/1932). However, in everyday practice, good reflection requires continual reevaluation of the process in light of findings along the way, even requiring the need to revisit prior considerations. For example, in reflecting on possible answers to a previously determined CEQ, it might be decided that the problem is, in fact, defined incorrectly, and thus we must go back and rethink the CEQ(s). (Examples can easily be multiplied in order to show any or all parts of the reflective process may need revisiting.)

WORKS CITED

Buermeyer, L., et al. 1923. *An introduction to reflective thinking*. Houghton Mifflin.
Dewey, J. 1910/1932. *How we think*. Heath and Co.

3

Reasoning in Ethics

Nancy S. Jecker

KEY POINTS

1. "Ethical relativism" is the view that the truth or falsity of ethical statements is relative to the culture of the person making the ethical statement.
2. One of the central arguments in support of ethical relativism is based on the observation that different cultures have different moral beliefs.
3. "Considered judgments" are judgments made when our moral capacities are most likely to be displayed without distortion.
4. "Principlism" is a method of ethical reasoning that draws upon ethical principles to lend support to practical decisions.
5. "Casuistry" is a method of ethical reasoning that helps us think about ethically uncertain situations by thinking about analogous cases and their associated maxims.
6. "Narrative ethics" is a method of ethical reasoning that uses fictional stories to engage critical thinking. For example, narrative ethics may use stories to show how moral choices and rules play out in the lives of fictional characters.

Public discussion of bioethics often arises in the context of particular cases. Most recently, the public debated what ought to be done in the case of Terri Schiavo, a woman in a persistent vegetative state whose husband requested removal of artificial nutrition and hydration, but whose parents insisted that everything possible be done to keep their daughter alive. Such discussion, which is motivated by practical exigencies and the need to make real decisions, often occurs in the absence of sustained reflection on underlying concepts and values. For example, rather than focusing on the concept of medical futility, or the principle of respect for patient autonomy, debate about the Schiavo case focused instead on the choices at hand: should health care providers stop or continue artificial nutrition and hydration? Similarly, listening to debates about therapeutic cloning or "partial birth" abortion, one hears little reference to the underlying philosophical concept of a "person." Instead, the focus is on deciding, for example, whether the law should or should not allow such practices.

Related to this is the fact that public bioethics debates tend to divide, rather than bring together, the different sides on an issue. In discussions of abortion, for example, not only does there appear to be no compromise position, there also is a phenomenon of digging in one's heels, that is, clinging tenaciously to one's own way of thinking while becoming closed to other viewpoints. For example, when appeal to religious or cultural values is made, these sources tend to function as conversation stoppers. In other words, a particular religious or cultural value tends to be presented as final or authoritative, rather than subject to interpretation and reasoned debate.

In light of this approach, which can be characterized as concrete and one-sided, it should come as no surprise that when laypeople enter the clinical setting of medicine, they are often unaware of how ethical decisions are made there. Specifically, they may show little awareness of how healthcare professionals think through ethical decisions and arrive at ethics recommendations. Because ethics methodologies are not widely known, there may be a tendency to assume that there are no methods of ethical analysis, and, correspondingly, no "right answer" to ethically controversial situations. In other words, there may be a tendency to assume that there are different points of view about ethical issues, each one equally valid. This view may also be a natural outcome of the concrete approach noted above, an approach that avoids delving beyond the surface of practical moral problems to the ethical values and ideas that underlie them.

Not only are laypeople sometimes unclear or confused about ethics, health professionals themselves may question how they do what they do, and what the source of their authority is. After all, most of a physician's or nurse's time is spent dealing with the practical concerns of clinicians and patients, not with discussing the methods and principles of ethics.

This chapter asks, To what extent is there a "method" for making ethical decisions? What role, if any, do theories and principles play in the justification of particular ethical decisions? Are the recommendations that hospital ethics committees (HECs) and ethics consultants offer backed by ethical argument, or do they merely reflect what is accepted as the norm by a given community? This chapter takes on the task of addressing these questions. It begins by considering the position that ethical judgments have no independent foundation, but are instead determined by what a particular group believes at a particular time. I point out the pitfalls of this approach, and move on to address the question of how ethical claims might be justified. Among the approaches I consider are principlism, casuistry, and narrative ethics. These approaches are not intended to be an exhaustive account of all available methods, but instead they are used for illustrative purposes. It is also fair to say that they represent some of the more common methodologies at work "behind the scenes" when ethicists and others assist with ethically difficult decisions. The goal throughout this chapter is to make approaches that foster critical thinking in ethics more widely known.

IS ETHICS RELATIVE?

We recognize that morality differs in every society, and it is a convenient term for socially approved habits. Mankind has always preferred to say, "It is a morally good," rather than "It is habitual," and the fact of this preference is matter enough for a critical science of ethics. But. . . the two phrases are synonymous. (Benedict 2006, 53)

Why start by considering the idea that "ethics is relative?" Clearly many people reject this idea and do not feel compelled to consider it further. The reason I begin here is that we live in an increasingly diverse society. Even if we are persuaded of the truth of our own moral beliefs, in the health care setting we must come to terms with the fact that we care for patients in multicultural contexts. This has not always been the case. During the first half of the twentieth century, most immigrants arriving on U.S. shores were Caucasians with European ancestry who shared the Judeo-Christian religion and traditions that were dominant in the United States at that time. However, during the second half of the twentieth century, and continuing today, many more immigrants come from the Far East and Middle East. They bring with them moral traditions and religious values, such as those of Islam, Shintoism, and Buddhism, that are dissimilar from the Judeo-Christian tradition. No longer can we assume that we all share the same ethical values and principles. We must instead tackle the question of whether we are ever justified in applying one group's values to another group. This question leads to another, namely: Are one group's moral beliefs any better than another group's? To address this, we need to look directly at the philosophical position of ethical relativism. It is to this task that I now turn.

We often hear the claim that "ethics is relative." There are moral truths, in other words, but they are relative to something. The problem with this type of claim is that it is terribly vague. It raises the further question, "relative to what?" Clearly there are several different things that ethical statements could be "relative" to. Thus, the truth or falsity of an ethical claim might be

1. relative to circumstances,
2. relative to a particular individual, or
3. relative to a particular culture.

Let us begin with the first interpretation. This is the view that (1) the truth or falsity of an ethical statement depends upon the *circumstances* that surround a particular case. Expressed differently, there are no "universal moral truths," that is, no ethical statements that are true in all situations. This idea is incorporated into diverse moral philosophies, such as situation ethics (Fletcher 1966) and act utilitarianism (Smart 1973), among others. This view rejects ethical absolutism, which holds that ethical rules and principles are the same regardless of the circumstances at hand. According to the absolutist, if lying is wrong, then it is always wrong to lie regardless of the circumstances. By contrast, someone who regards the truth or falsity of ethical statements as circumstance-bound allows for the possibility that whether lying is right or wrong may vary, depending upon the circumstances of the particular case.

Notice that the position that ethics is relative to the circumstances of a particular case leaves open the possibility of justifying moral claims by appealing to standards that hold circumstantially, yet are independent of what a particular culture or individual believes. One might, for example, hold that lying is wrong whenever certain circumstances are present, independent of what particular individuals or cultures believe. Therefore a person can accept the first view, namely, that ethics is (1) relative to circumstances, yet reject the second or third views, which hold that ethics is (2) relative to a particular individual or (3) relative to a culture.

Consider next the claim that the truth or falsity of ethical statements is (2) relative to a particular individual. This view, which is called "ethical subjectivism," suggests that ethical terms are expressions of the speaker's subjective state, for example, the speaker's attitudes or beliefs. The ethical subjectivist maintains that moral claims are indeed true and false, yet their truth or falsity depends solely upon the subjective state of the person making the claim. So, for example, if someone says that "abortion is wrong," this claim is true for that individual if she believes that abortion is wrong or has a negative attitude toward abortion, and false otherwise.

Finally, to say that ethics is relative to (3) a particular culture suggests something quite different. It suggests that the truth or falsity of ethical sentences depends upon the *culture* of the person making the claim. This view, which is properly referred to as "ethical relativism," holds that each culture has its own moral code, and all moral codes have an equal claim to validity. In other words, there is no standard external to all cultures by which the ethical code of particular cultures can be judged.

The position that ethics is relative to circumstances will be investigated below in the context of talking about the methods of casuistry and narrative ethics. For now I set this position aside. The once powerful view known as ethical subjectivism I will also set aside. When it first emerged during the 1940s and 1950s, and was popularized by philosophers such as A. J. Ayer (1952), C. L. Stevenson (1944), and R. M. Hare (1952), it was widely criticized. It is fair to say that today it has been largely discredited (Arrington 1989). This leaves us with the position of ethical relativism. Ethical relativism continues to be discussed in the scholarly literature (Wong 1984), and its influence has only increased with the controversies raised by multicultural critiques of Western values, which assert that traditional ethics is biased in favor of Western culture (Sterba 2001). Therefore, it is to this third view that I now turn.

MOTIVES UNDERLYING ETHICAL RELATIVISM

There are a variety of motivations that lead people to accept ethical relativism. One motive is the practical experience of trying to resolve very difficult ethical problems. After a while, one may begin to feel that there must not be any answer if one cannot be found or agreed upon. Generalizing this, one might be led to think that this is simply the "nature" of ethical problems. In other words, one might conclude that answers to ethical questions cannot be found because ethical statements have no justification outside of what a particular person or group believes.

Yet despite the initial attraction of this approach, it is difficult to sustain upon reflection. After all, in many other areas of thought the answers to questions may be difficult to discern, yet it hardly follows that there is no right answer, or that answers depend solely on what an individual or group believes. For example, a group of preschoolers presented with the question, "What is seven minus two?" may each come up with different answers. Yet it hardly follows that there is no right answer to this question, or that all answers are equally valid. Similarly, physicists may find it difficult to describe the smallest particles of matter, but it hardly follows that there is no true description, or that all descriptions are equally correct. Analogously, it may be difficult to settle an ethical controversy, yet it hardly follows that there is no right answer, or that every answer is equally valid.

Another motive leading people to embrace ethical relativism begins with the observation that we typically regard toleration for diverse views as a virtue. It might be thought that embracing ethical relativism will encourage developing this virtue. For example, we would naturally show greater respect for people whose views differed from our own if we regarded their views as equally valid, rather than "wrong." Likewise, we would show greater humility about our own values, and less arrogance toward others, if we held the belief that all values have equal standing.

However, in response to this approach, opponents of ethical relativism point out that although toleration of diverse views is a virtue, this virtue has limits. For example, opponents of ethical relativism think in terms of a society that mistreats certain groups, or is wantonly cruel to innocent people, and insists on condemning this. Susan Okin, for example, calls attention to the fact that many culturally based practices aim to control women or render them servile to men's desires and interests (Okin 1999). She claims that when a non-Western culture resists assimilation to Western liberal values and asserts group rights as a means of holding on to patriarchal values, this should not be tolerated. Instead, our response should be to assert that women and men are moral equals, and sex discrimination is wrong.

ARGUMENTS SUPPORTING ETHICAL RELATIVISM

Motivations aside, what are the strongest arguments in favor of ethical relativism? One of the most common arguments comes from social science disciplines, such as anthropology. It begins with the observation that careful study of the practices of different cultural groups supports the idea that what is and is not behaviorally "normal" is culturally determined. In a similar fashion, it is reasoned that what is ethically right and wrong is also culturally determined. This argument can be formulated more precisely as follows (Benedict 2006, 49–54):

1. Different cultures have radically different practices.
2. Therefore different cultures have different moral codes.
3. Therefore one culture's moral code is no better than any other culture's moral code.

In response, it can be pointed out that this argument encounters many difficulties. First, the second premise claims to follow from the first premise, yet clearly premise one could be true, but premise two false. In other words, societies that tolerate different practice may in fact agree about fundamental moral principles. Two different cultures may agree, for example, about the principle that one should respect the dead. Yet this principle may be expressed in radically different ways, with one culture showing respect for the dead by burning the dead, and another culture showing respect for the dead by eating the dead. There are different practices for sure, but no differences in the underlying ethical principles to which each group is committed. In conclusion, in order for ethical relativists to draw support from the fact of moral diversity, they must be able to show that different moral practices reflect different underlying values.

A second difficulty this argument faces is that the conclusion purports to follow from the second premise, yet premise two could be true and the conclusion false. To see that this is so, consider an analogy. Throughout history, different societies have held different scientific beliefs. Therefore, one scientific belief is no better than any other. Yet clearly this is false. It is false to say that Ptolemy's view that the earth is the center of the universe is no better than Copernicus's view that the sun is the center of the universe. This analogy serves to make the broader point that differences of opinion about a topic can indicate many things, and do not necessarily establish that opposing views are equally valid. Nor does disagreement establish that there is no truth about a particular matter. Instead, the burden of proof is on the ethical relativist to demonstrate that the same act is both right and wrong, or that the same ethical principle is both true and false.

These difficulties aside, the central objection to this argument is that it moves from purely descriptive claims, in the premises, to a normative claim, in the conclusion. Yet this inference from empirical to normative claims is hardly valid. At best, a descriptive claim can lend inductive support to a more general descriptive claim. For example after seeing a hundred white swans and no swans that are not white, I may conclude, "All swans are white." Yet my observations do not support any nonempirical claim about swans, such as that "All swans should be white," or "White swans are better than swans of other colors."

A second argument frequently cited in support of ethical relativism begins by noting that many beliefs and practices, including some moral beliefs and practices, are simply conventions of the culture. Thus, it might be thought that this is true of moral claims more generally. This argument, which some date back to the fifth-century B.C. historian, Herodotus, can be expressed in the following way (Herodotus 1986):

1. Whether it is ethically right to *do some specific act* (e.g., burn or eat the dead) depends upon the culture from which one is born.
2. Therefore, the truth or falsity of *all* ethical statements is relative to the culture to which a person belongs.

Yet in response it can be said that if this argument is understood as an inductive argument (which means that the premise lends some support to the conclusion but does not prove that the conclusion is true), it is rather weak. Alternatively, considered as a deductive argument (where the conclusion is said to follow with necessity if the premises are true), it is not valid. That is, one can accept the premise, yet deny the conclusion. One could certainly agree that there is no culturally independent ethical standard to judge how we ought to treat the dead, yet still hold that there is a culturally independent standard for judging other ethical claims. Indeed many areas of morality may be culturally determined, yet it does not follow that *all* areas of ethics are culturally determined. Someone who supports the position defined as "ethical relativism" needs to establish not just that the truth or falsity of *some* ethical statement is culturally determined, but instead that the truth or falsity of *all* ethical statements are culturally determined.

Finally, in support of relativism, it is often argued that different ethical claims must be equally valid because there is no generally agreed-upon foundation or basis for a universally binding moral code (Stace 1986).

1. If there is a universally binding moral code, then there must be some foundation or basis for such a code. In other words, "a command implies a commander," or "an obligation implies an authority which obliges."
2. We have not yet found an acceptable foundation upon which a universal moral code can be based.
3. Therefore, there is no universally binding moral code.

The response to this argument was already established above; namely, the absence of agreement about some matter does not establish that all views are equally valid. In this case, the absence of agreement about the foundation for a universal morality does not suffice to show that there is no such foundation. There may be a valid basis for a universally binding moral code that has not yet been recognized or accepted.

METHODS OF ETHICAL REASONING

If the above reasoning is sound, then some of the most common motives and reasons people have for favoring ethical relativism do not withstand careful scrutiny. Clearly, more could be said about the question of ethical relativism, and about the broader question of how ethical claims are justified. For now, however, let us set these questions

aside, and move forward with the assumption that it is possible to justify ethical claims. Let us assume further that the justification of ethical claims is not based on the beliefs or attitudes of the individual
making the claim (ethical subjectivism), or on the culture of the person making the claim (ethical relativism). Instead, let us assert that
reason provides the necessary tools for justification and let us consider
how one would go about appealing to reason to justify moral claims.
This brings us back to the question with which we began, namely:
what methods of ethical analysis and argument are used in clinical settings to support ethical judgments in particular cases?

In clinical settings, health professionals and ethicists employ a variety of tools of critical analysis. Before delving into these, it is helpful to first step back and introduce a more general way of thinking
about ethical reasoning. This way of thinking has as its starting point
the idea of a "considered judgment." According to Rawls, considered
judgments are

> judgments in which our moral capacities are most likely to be dis-
> played without distortion. . . . Considered judgments are simply
> those rendered . . . where the more common excuses and explana-
> tions for making a mistake do not obtain. . . . [T]he criteria . . . are
> not arbitrary. They are, in fact, similar to those that single out consid-
> ered judgments of any kind. . . . [T]he relevant judgments are those
> given under conditions favorable for deliberation and judgment in
> general. (Rawls 1971, 48)

The suggestion is that we discard moral judgments made with hesitation, or in which we have little confidence, as well as those given
when we are upset or frightened, or when we stand to gain one way
or the other. Such judgments are likely to be erroneous, or to be biased in favor of our own interests.

Once established, our "considered judgments" about particular
moral situations can function as the "facts" that our ethical principles and theories must match. The goal of requiring our principles
and theories to match our considered judgment is to arrive, ultimately, at a state Rawls calls "reflective equilibrium" (Rawls 1971,
20). Reflective equilibrium is a state of "equilibrium," because our
practical judgments and ethical principles coincide, rather than conflict, with each another. It is "reflective," because we know the principles to which our judgments conform, and the premises of their

derivation. To arrive at reflective equilibrium, we first form carefully considered judgments about particular cases. Next, we determine the ethical principles that these judgments evince (which may require simply identifying an already established principle, or may require more, for example, developing a new principle to apply to the case). Ultimately, establishing a state of harmony between practical judgments and general moral principles requires revising either our judgments or our principles, or both. So understood, reflective equilibrium is not a stable state, because it is liable to be upset as new moral dilemmas present themselves, challenging our ethical beliefs and principles anew.

The ideas of considered judgments and reflective equilibrium lay a groundwork for understanding how diverse methods of ethical decision making assist with the process of critical reflection. In choosing a method of ethical analysis and applying it to a case, the goal is both pragmatic and philosophical. Pragmatically, we want to engage critical thinking about the case and reach a decision about what to do. Philosophically, we want to align practical clinical decisions and fundamental values and reach a state of harmony and "equilibrium" among our beliefs.

Principlism

Let us turn next to look at three ethical methodologies that fit well with the Rawlsian framework just laid out. The first approach, known as "principlism," engages critical thinking about cases by calling upon ethical principles to lend support to practical decisions. Principlism, which is associated with philosophers Tom Beauchamp and James Childress, typically draws upon four principles, which it is claimed derive authority from considered judgments in common morality and medical traditions. The four principles can be stated as follows.

1. *Principle of Respect for Autonomy*: One ought to respect the autonomous choices of persons.
2. *Principle of Beneficence*: One ought to do good, and prevent or remove harm.
3. *Principle of Nonmaleficence*: One ought to refrain from inflicting harm.
4. *Principle of Justice*: One ought to treat equals equally.

Principlism holds that particular ethical judgments are justified by showing that they follow from one of these four ethical principles, and that the principles themselves match our considered judgments. For example, we justify the particular claim that artificial nutrition and hydration should be removed from a person in a persistent vegetative state by (1) appealing to the principle of respect for autonomy and (2) citing the patient's living will, which directs physicians not to use any life-sustaining treatments, including artificial nutrition and hydration, in the event that the patient is diagnosed as being in a persistent vegetative state.

It is important to note that principlism allows for the possibility that reaching reflective equilibrium may require revising our considered judgments about either a particular case or a general moral principle (Beauchamp and Childress 2001, 398). According to principlism, the ultimate support for ethical claims is not principles per se, but considered judgments. In other words, ethics is ultimately grounded on those moral judgments about which we have the highest degree of confidence. For example, we hold a high degree of confidence about the following general claims:

1. Racial discrimination is wrong.
2. Religious intolerance is wrong.
3. Political repression is wrong.

Notice too that we also have a high degree of confidence about more specific claims, such as the following:

4. The institution of slavery in the American South was wrong.
5. The persecution of Jews during World War II was wrong.
6. The repression of political dissent in the former Soviet Union was wrong.

Thus, considered judgments can occur at any level of generality, from the most particular to the most general. It would be misleading to characterize principlism as a view that concrete ethical judgments are justified by appealing to more general ethical principles. This is because both particular judgments and general moral principles must withstand the test of our considered judgments. For example, the principle of beneficence in medicine came to be seen as limited in scope, especially during the 1960s and 1970s when there was a growing awareness of the value of respect for patient autonomy. Or, to take another example, the principle of autonomy came to be seen as limited in scope, especially during the 1990s when justice-based challenges called attention to the fact that societies have a finite amount of money to spend on health care. In summary, both particular judgments and general moral principles may be altered to match our considered judgments. In this manner, we aim to achieve equilibrium, thereby bringing all of our moral beliefs into a coherent whole that matches our most firmly held moral convictions.

Casuistry

Let us turn next to consider a second approach to ethical analysis. This approach, known as casuistry, differs from principlism because it calls our attention first and foremost to the particular facts of each individual case. Casuistry engages critical thinking about cases by asking us to find and consider analogous cases, that is, cases that are similar in morally relevant respects. To facilitate case comparison, the casuist organizes cases on the basis of "paradigm" cases. A "paradigm" is a case that presents a relatively clear and simple moral situation. Cases that move away from a paradigm introduce specific circumstances that make the moral situation more obscure or complex. Cases can be organized into a kind of taxonomy, beginning with those that present the most clear and simple moral dilemmas (the paradigms) and then introducing specific circumstances that depart from the paradigm in specific ways.

Associated with each paradigm is a "maxim" or well-established moral principle that provides warrant or justification for the expert opinion about the case. Maxims have a variety of sources. Albert Jonsen and Stephen Toulmin (1988, 253), for example, cite maxims, such as "force may be repulsed by force" and "defense measured to the need of the occasion," which are based on Roman law, as well as maxims, such as "don't kick a man when he is down," which reflect what ordinary people might say when arguing about a moral issue.

As noted already, cases that move away from a paradigm display complicating circumstances. "Circumstances" include features such as who, what, where, when, why, how, and by what means. For instance, a patient with decisional capacity may choose to forego prescribed chemotherapy and radiation following a diagnosis of breast cancer. She may opt instead for mastectomy alone. The maxim in such a case could be expressed as the injunction that a patient with decisional capacity has a right to refuse any treatment. Analogous cases of treatment refusal may draw upon this paradigm case and its associated maxim. For example, in an analogous case, a patient in a persistent vegetative state may have left clear and convincing evidence, in the form of a directive to physicians, stating that he would not want to be kept alive on a ventilator under such circumstances. The fact that the patient is unconscious and unable to speak for himself is a circumstance that renders the case less clear and convincing than the paradigm. Additional complicating circumstances might include, for example, that the patient has not left any clear statement of wishes, or family members disagree about what the patient would want, or the diagnosis of persistent vegetative state is disputed. Such circumstances make it successively more difficult to apply the maxim associated with the paradigm without qualifying or modifying it to fit the circumstances of the new case.

As this example attests, casuistry requires heightened sensitivity to the differences and similarities among cases. In this sense, one could say that casuistry suggests that "ethics is relative," not to the individual or cultural group, but to the circumstances of a particular case. Casuistry maintains that the general maxims of morality apply to certain types of cases in certain types of circumstances. As we move away from these, casuistry requires us to modify our maxims. Historically, casuistry took on its modern, pejorative meaning only when its maxims became "generalized and exaggerated," that is, no longer embedded within particular cases and circumstances (Jonsen and Toulmin 1988, 255).

Casuistry displays a methodological kinship with the approach of reflective equilibrium discussed above. Just as Rawls (1971) distinguishes between moral judgments where there is a high degree of certainty (considered judgments), and those where there is less certainty, so too the casuist qualifies moral judgments about cases in terms of their "probability." According to casuistry, the cases and associated maxims that display the highest degree of probability are the paradigms. As we move from paradigms to analogous cases, and from maxims associated with paradigms to slightly modified maxims associated with analogous cases, we introduce increasing degrees of complexity and uncertainty.

Just as Rawls (1971) stresses consistency among moral beliefs, so casuists stress the need to make comparisons among analogous cases so that moral judgments are consistent across cases. Likewise, casuists require placing general maxims in the context of particular cases, so that general and particular judgments are brought into harmony. In the end, casuistry (like Rawlsian reflective equilibrium) requires revising both general maxims and particular judgments to match our most certain beliefs. According to casuistry, judgments gain certainty when attached to clear and simple cases (paradigms). So understood, generalized maxims do not posses in isolation either a high or low "probability." Instead the certainty of maxims is pragmatically based, that is, determined by how well maxims function in particular cases. Thus, the highest degree of certainty applies to maxims that have been successfully tested and fine-tuned in a large number of cases. For example, the maxim that asserts patients have a "right to privacy" or a "right to determine what happens in and to their bodies" has been tested and fine-tuned in a large number of cases, dating back to paradigms, such as Karen Quinlan and *Roe v. Wade*. While it continues to be debated and its application to new situations, such as Oregon's Death with Dignity Act, remains highly controversial, the maxim that we "own our bodies" and have a right to privacy has gained a relatively high degree of confidence. A maxim achieves this status in light of an accumulation of cases, which represent a kind of cumulative argument for the maxim. Summarizing this point, Jonsen and Toulmin compare casuistical argument to

the rhetorical and commonsense discourse that piles up many kinds of argument in hopes of showing the favored position in good light. The "weight" of a casuistical opinion came from the accumulation of reasons rather than from the logical validity of the arguments or the coherence of any single "proof." (Jonsen and Toulmin 1988, 256)

Narrative Ethics

A third and final approach to ethical argument and analysis is narrative ethics. Narrative ethics is variously interpreted. This position might be interpreted as the view that encourages us to see patients as more than merely "cases" and associated medical diagnoses, but also as persons with narrative histories and meanings who must try to fit disease and disability into their own life story. So understood, narrative techniques assist healthcare providers to understand and respond to patients in richer, more meaningful ways (Hunter 1991). A related approach, proposed by physician and literary scholar Rita

Charon, encourages health professionals to develop "narrative competence" to improve their understanding of and connection with patients (Charon 2004, 862–64). A somewhat different interpretation of narrative ethics, from Nina Rosenstand, encourages us to use fictional stories like a lab, where ethical principles can be "experimented with" or applied to moral issues under controlled conditions (Rosenstand 2003, vii).

All of these interpretations of narrative ethics are consistent with the idea that narrative ethics is as a mode of ethical analysis that leaves intact the basic structure of principle-based accounts, and sees narrative techniques as a supplement to principles (Arras 1997, 65–88). All of these accounts share with casuistry a focus on concrete situations, although narrative ethics, unlike casuistry, uses works of fiction. Whereas casuistry judges what to do in particular cases by comparing cases to moral paradigms, narrative ethics may render moral judgments in a variety of ways.

First, narrative approaches may invite us to think about how moral decisions play out in the lives of fictional characters. For example, in thinking about a fictional story, we may be led to ask, How might this person's life have been different if she had made a different moral choice? Or, after observing characters over the course of a story, readers may be asked, What about this character do I admire? What do I dislike or disapprove of? Thinking critically about fictional characters can help us to think more carefully about actual people and role models in real life.

Second, narrative ethics may judge moral rules and codes of conduct by using stories to teach and question them. For example, narrative approaches take stories that express a moral point of view, and then question and discuss that point of view. The value of seeing moral rules or viewpoints in narrative context, rather than in abstraction, is that we can potentially appreciate better what it means to follow certain rules or viewpoints. For example, we can observe how a rule, such as "tell the truth," plays out over the course of a story in the lives of fictional characters. Moral rules and codes can thus be investigated in the context of an entire way of life.

Finally, narrative approaches may encourage us to judge other people's lives and choices empathically. Narrative approaches use stories to foster empathy by enabling readers to live vicariously the lives of fictional characters. For example, medical students who consider not only medical cases, but also stories of fiction, such as Leo

Tolstoy's *The Death of Ivan Ilyich*, are potentially better able to appreciate a patient's point of view. At the same time, however, when stories have an emotional impact, narrative approaches stress combining our emotional responses to a story with reasoning about our emotions. As Rosenstand points out, "Feelings can be manipulated, and appeals to emotions don't solve [moral] conflicts," because different people may feel differently about a situation (Rosenstand 2003, 13).

Like the methods of principlism and casuistry discussed above, narrative methods encourage exploring moral beliefs in a careful and systematic way. When stories are used to engage critical thinking, they help us to form more considered judgments about moral situations. By investigating a variety of stories that present different points of view on a moral issue, for example, we can appreciate moral controversies more fully. While narrative ethics does not emphasize the Rawlsian idea of arriving at a state of harmony or equilibrium among all of our moral beliefs, presumably it can help with this as well. After all, just as casuistry employs cases to develop a cumulative argument for a particular maxim, so too can narrative approaches use multiple stories to lend increasing support to a particular moral lesson or way of life. Moreover, as suggested already, narrative ethics sometimes uses stories in tandem with moral principles, allowing the stories to function like "tests" for moral principles and theories. This strategy enables us to check and make sure that our general moral beliefs are in harmony with our particular moral judgments.

CONCLUSION

I began this chapter by asking a series of questions, so let us return to these questions and see what answers are forthcoming. The first question was, Is there a method for making ethical decisions? Our discussion makes evident that a variety of established methods exist to facilitate critical thinking in ethics. These approaches draw on different kinds of ethical reasoning to assess moral choices or resolve moral uncertainty. The tendency, discussed above, to think that ethical judgments are based solely on what an individual or culture believes is, at first blush, not persuasive. Instead, systematic approaches for examining moral beliefs enable us to think critically about what individuals and groups believe.

I also asked, What role, if any, do ethical theories and principles play in the justification of particular ethical decisions? The short answer to this question is that ethical principles and the theories with which they are associated play an important role in the justification of ethical decisions. The longer answer is that the exact role they play depends, in part, upon which among several methods of ethical analysis a person uses. For example, the approach of principlism clearly directs us to consider the ethical principles that underlie and justify a particular point of view. According to principlism, however, ethical principles are themselves subject to revision, and they derive authority from our considered judgments about both particular cases and more general moral beliefs. Thus the ultimate justification of ethical claims is not principles per se, but considered judgments themselves.

By contrast, casuistry asks us to compare our immediate situation of moral uncertainty to an analogous case where there is a more settled opinion. Thus ethical reflection begins with reviewing the particular circumstances of a case and comparing it to a case with analogous circumstances. Yet principles also come into play at other stages of deliberation, for example, where they are incorporated into the "settled opinion" or "maxims" associated with a paradigm case. For example, the principle of autonomy might come into play in a casuistic analysis of the case of Terri Schiavo discussed above, because this principle is incorporated into the settled opinion of other paradigm cases, such as Nancy Cruzan (Jonsen, Veatch, and Walters 1998a, 229–37) and Karen Quinlan (Jonsen, Veatch, and Walters 1998b, 143–48).

Like casuistry, narrative approaches invoke cases, but these cases are fictional accounts, typically longer and more detailed than the usual case presentation. Like casuistry, narrative approaches do not necessarily reject ethical principles. Rather, narrative ethics may use stories to evaluate and "test" moral principles by placing them in narrative context so that we can appreciate better what it means to live by a certain principle. On this interpretation, principles themselves remain a critical component of ethical analysis.

Finally, I asked at the outset whether the recommendations of ethics committees and ethics consultants were backed by ethical argument, or merely reflect what is accepted by the norm by a given community. In response it can be said that in the clinical setting, moral controversies are increasingly dealt with by utilizing the kinds of systematic approaches described here. The requirements of the Joint Commission for the Accreditation of Health Care Organizations (JCAHO) requires hospitals and other institutions receiving federal funding to have ethics committees. The role of HECs is designed to ensure that ethical decisions and policies undergo review, are arrived at through a fair process, and are publicly accountable. Clearly the recommendations of HECs and ethics consultants reflect the norms of the healthcare professions, but these norms are critically discussed and interpreted using a process of rational deliberation. This process can no doubt be improved through greater utilization of quality assurance techniques, such as ethics training for HEC members and retrospective review of ethics consultation services.

I also began this chapter with examples of moral cases and policies that sparked public debate and controversy. I pointed out that these debates are often one-sided and concrete, and I promised to offer some ways of thinking more carefully about difficult moral choices. All of the methods discussed in this chapter enable us to move beyond the particular case at hand and to think in a more general way about the values at stake in a situation. All of the methods introduced here help us to move outside of our own way of thinking and explore other viewpoints. Finally, all of the methods discussed here employ the language of reason, rather than the strategy of digging in our heels, in an effort to reach moral consensus with others. By making these methods of ethical analysis more widely known, ethicists (and others) can encourage reasoned debate about ethically problematic situations. This benefits patients and families in the clinical setting and helps all of us in the broader moral community.

FOR FURTHER REFLECTION

1. What is ethical relativism? How does it differ from other views that hold "ethics is relative?"
2. What is the strongest argument you can think of in support of ethical relativism? Does this argument succeed? Why or why not?
3. What is "reflective equilibrium?" What role do "considered judgments" play in the process of establishing reflective equilibrium?
4. Name three methods of ethical reasoning. How are they similar? How are they different?

5. What is a "paradigm," and what role do paradigms play in casuistry?
6. When ethical principles conflict with judgments about a particular case, what means of resolution is open to someone who endorses the method known as "principlism?"

WORKS CITED

Arras, J. 1997. Nice story, but so what? In *Stories and their limits*, ed. H. Lindemann Nelson, 65–88. New York: Routledge.

Arrington, R. L. 1989. *Rationalism, realism, and relativism: Perspectives in contemporary moral epistemology*. Ithaca, NY: Cornell University Press.

Ayer, A. J. 1952. *Language, truth and logic*. New York: Dover.

Beauchamp, T. L., and J. F. Childress. 2001. *Principles of biomedical ethics*, 5th ed. New York: Oxford University Press.

Benedict, R. 2006. A defense of ethical relativism. Reprinted in *Conduct and character: Readings in moral theory*, 5th ed., ed. Mark Timmons. Belmont, CA: Thomson Wadsworth.

Charon, R. 2004. Narrative and medicine. *New England Journal of Medicine* 350 (9): 862–64.

Fletcher, J. 1966. *Situation ethics: The new morality*. Philadelphia: Westminster.

Hare, R. M. 1952. *The language of morals*. New York: Oxford University Press.

Herodotus. 1986. Morality as custom. Reprinted in *Right and wrong: Basic readings in ethics*, ed. C. Hoff Sommers, 132–33. San Diego, CA: Harcourt, Brace, Jovanovich.

Hunter, K. M. 1991. *Doctors' stories: The narrative structure of medical knowledge*. Princeton, NJ: Princeton University Press.

Jonsen, A. R., and S. Toulmin. 1988. *The abuse of casuistry*. Berkeley, CA: University of California Press.

Jonsen, A. R., R. M. Veatch, L. Walters, eds. 1998a. *Cruzan v. Director, Missouri Department of Health*: U.S. Supreme Court. In *Source book in bioethics: A documentary history*, 229–37. Washington, DC: Georgetown University Press.

———, eds. 1998b. *In the Matter of Karen Quinlan*: The Supreme Court, State of New Jersey. In *Source book in bioethics: A documentary history*, 143–48. Washington, DC: Georgetown University Press.

Okin, S. M. 1999. Is multiculturalism bad for women? In *Is multiculturalism bad for women?*, ed. S. M. Okin, 9–24. Princeton, NJ: Princeton University Press.

Rawls, J. 1971. *A theory of justice*. Cambridge, MA: Harvard University Press.

Rosenstand, N., ed. 2003. *The moral of the story*, 4th ed. Boston: McGraw Hill.

Smart, J. C. C. 1973. An outline of a system of utilitarian ethics. In *Utilitarianism: For and against*, ed. J. J. C. Smart and B. Williams. New York: Cambridge University Press.

Stace, W. T. 1986. Ethical relativism: A critique. Reprinted in *Right and wrong: Basic readings in ethics*, ed. C. Hoff Sommers, 142–55. San Diego, CA: Harcourt, Brace, Jovanovich.

Sterba, J. P. 2001. The western bias in traditional ethics and how to correct it. In *Three challenges to ethics: Environmentalism, feminism, and multiculturalism*, 77–103. New York: Oxford University Press.

Stevenson, C. L. 1944. *Ethics and language*. New Haven, CT: Yale University Press.

Wong, D. 1984. *Moral relativity*. Berkeley, CA: University of California Press.

4

Ethics Consultation and the Committee

Wayne Shelton and Dyrleif Bjarnadottir

KEY POINTS

1. Discuss the kinds of ethical conflicts in cases that require ethics consultation.
2. Describe the steps involved in performing a clinical ethics consultation.
3. Consider the qualifications and skills necessary to work as an ethics consultant.
4. Explain the various models and approaches used in ethics consultations.

During the past four decades, we have witnessed increasing medical knowledge and technology, along with the growing awareness of the range of diverse needs and wishes of the patient population (Lo 1987; Hollinger 1989; Fletcher and Hoffman 1994; Sugarman 1994; Kelly 2004). As a result, clinical ethical dilemmas have become more complex, and the need to address them in a manner that involves special expertise ever more apparent. Not surprisingly, ethics consultation has become a common and widely accepted practice in U.S. hospitals, with 86 percent of hospital ethics committees (HECs) reporting that they play a role in ongoing clinical decision making through clinical ethics consultation (McGee et al. 2001).

HECs are typically charged with the responsibilities of overseeing, doing, or participating in ethics consultations. As such, members should understand basic information about the ethics consultation process. There is no doubt that such tasks can be daunting for HEC members; in fact, they may be the most daunting of all HEC tasks—as often, direct and identifiable patient care is at issue. Although most members have clinical experience, they often lack formal educational training in clinical ethics and ethics consultation, but what kind of tools, knowledge, and expertise do they need actually need?

This chapter will provide HEC members with some basic practical information to guide them in their oversight of, and possible participation in, ethics consultations. Specifically, this chapter is intended to provide HEC members a basis for answering and exploring further the following questions:

- What kinds of cases are referred to an ethics consultation service?
- What are the steps in the process and methodology of an ethics consultation?
- What kinds of expertise and qualifications are necessary to do ethics consultations?
- What are the models of ethics consultation?
- What are the techniques used for conflict resolution?

We will begin with three case descriptions from our own ethics consultation service that represent the types of ethical issues often referred for ethics consultation.

CLINICAL CASES INVOLVING ETHICAL CONFLICT

Case #1

An eighty-six-year-old woman with a prior medical history of hypertension and congestive heart failure (CHF) fell from her wheelchair at her home while experiencing dizziness and lightheadedness. She was able to call emergency medical services (EMS) and was transported to the emergency department (ED). After ten days of hospitalization and being treated for a gastrointestinal (GI) bleed, which has resolved, she is now stable and no longer needs to be in the hospital. However, her caregivers feel that because she is wheelchair bound, she is too weak to make difficult transfers in her home where she lives alone. She does not have the resources nor is she inclined to hire a full-time caregiver. She is strongly advised by her hospital caregivers to spend a week or two in rehab before attempting to return home. They believe that for her to go back home now is setting her up for another fall or problem that will cause further harm to her and require hospitalizations. She refuses to go to rehab and insists on going home to resume her life of independence. Although she is very hard of hearing, she is alert and communicative.

Case #2

An eighty-year-old man was transferred from a nursing home to a local ED with excruciating belly pain. He was diagnosed to have a ruptured abdominal aortic aneurysm (AAA) and was in urgent need of surgical repair if he was to live. He was awake at the time and was reported to have given consent to have surgery; however, the patient was also on morphine sedation at that time. The patient was then transferred by helicopter to a regional medical center, where successful surgical repair of the AAA took place. The patient was then taken to the Surgical Intensive Care Unit (SICU). At present, the patient is unconscious and on life supports but stable, in critical condition. His survival is in question, but if he does survive, he faces long rehabilitation. His three sons, who have been out of town, now arrive at the SICU with the patient's living will and healthcare proxy document. They are all in agreement that he would not want the present treatment, and ask the attending physician to consider withdrawal of care.

Case #3

Mrs. P is a thirty-six-year-old woman, admitted to the oncology unit with end-stage metastatic cancer of the appendix. She was diagnosed with the cancer about nine months prior to this admission and received some chemotherapy, which was unsuccessful. She has also explored a number of alternative treatments, but they too have been unsuccessful. She and her husband are deeply religious Christians and have had faith that she would be miraculously cured. They have three elementary-school-aged children. In the week before she was admitted she had been steadily declining, and it seemed that her death was imminent. She was being taken care of by a hospice service at home, receiving total parenteral nutrition (TPN) and pain medication. Although she was awake at the time of her hospital admission, she appeared to be actively dying. She was emaciated, agitated, and unable to communicate and showed very limited mobility and sensory perception. She no longer had the capacity to speak for herself, and her husband was her primary decision maker. The husband's request for transfer to the local medical center was based on the claim that she needed better pain management. However, once she was admitted, he also requests that "we do everything" including CPR, intubation and ICU care. He claims that he is making requests for treatment based on his wife's expressed wishes.

_____ ◦∞∞◦ _____

In the above cases, the requests for an ethics consultation were based on the clinical caregivers' experiences in which they were engaged with patients and families concerning deep conflicts of value about the right course of action. In each case, physicians perceive their professional obligations to the patients are being called into question; and yet as human beings, physicians' own feelings, predispositions, and values influence their perspectives not only toward the features of the case and patient care, but toward the requests and interests of others. Their professional and personal responses to clinical cases can collide with preferences and values of patients and their families and friends. For example, Case #1 illustrates the beneficence-based obligation to take care of and protect a vulnerable patient over and against the patient's strong impulse to remain free and independent. Case #2, in turn, illustrates a perceived professional obligation to continue treatment and hope for a favorable medical outcome over and against the patient's wishes, being expressed by a loving family, to limit current and future medical burdens. Lastly, Case #3 illustrates the deep concern of a physician that the medical treatments being requested by the family may force her to violate her oath to do no harm. Each of these cases, and many types of cases that require ethics consultation, reflect value conflicts in what can be called a "problematic situation."

Problematic situations arise from a deep feeling of concern of one or more individuals in reaction to a state of affairs. This results in serious obstacles to the normal or assumed way of proceeding in a case, usually involving two or more conflicting value-laden points of view. Thus, until the problematic situation is addressed, direction and progress are stalled. There are ways out of the impasse, if the people involved are able to discuss and share their basic factual and moral assumptions, and remain open to explore and negotiate new options that are mutually agreeable. Although some conflicts become intractable and favorable outcomes difficult, a well-trained and skilled ethics consultant can facilitate, based on the unique features of the particular problematic situation, an outcome about which all parties involved are more comfortable (Hester 2001).

BACKGROUND AND EXPERTISE OF THE ETHICS CONSULTANT

HECs as consultants, thus, can be well situated with an institution to help open up conversation about values issues, to help identify the nature of values conflicts, and to help develop means of overcoming such conflicts. However, before discussing our methodology for providing such help through ethics consultations, it is important to consider the important challenge of who should be an ethics consultant in conflicts (like those in the above three cases). What are the qualifications of such an individual? What counts as expertise? In every hospital that has an ethics consultation service, these broad questions will need to be addressed in terms of a clear and practical hospital policy that fits each institutional setting.

These questions are not new, as there has been considerable debate from the early days of ethics consultation about the qualifications and expertise necessary to do them. These debates often turned on competing and sometimes confused understandings of the role of the ethics consultant (Yoder 1998). One prevalent source of misunderstanding has been the idea that ethicists are moral experts and provide substantive moral advice to physicians and nurses, that is, ethics experts can give the "right" answers just like other medical experts (Noble 1982; Scofield 1993). By the mid- to late 1990s, such characterizations were much less common as the field began to mature and agree upon the nature of its purpose. By 1998, there was an emerging consensus that the role of the ethics consultant was best described as one of ethics facilitation, which is

> fundamentally consistent with the rights of individuals to live by their own moral values by not displacing decision-making authority or acceding to the personal views of the consultant. . . and is consistent with the

rights of individuals to live by their own moral values and the fact of pluralism. (American Society for Bioethics and Humanities 1998)

Within the field, it should be a common assumption by now that
clinical ethics must be understood in the context of a democratic,
pluralistic society in which competing value positions can be heard.
Therefore, much of the expertise necessary to do clinical ethics consultations is connected with facilitating a process in which conflicts
are addressed according to well-established rights and obligations
inherent in the physician-patient relationship as well as being informed by law and institutional policy.

Even with this consensus concerning facilitation, ethics consultation
involves skills related to both ethical understanding and clinical experience. Thus, some debates have focused on what background provides the necessary expertise to do ethics consultations, particularly
pitting a philosophical background against that of clinical medicine—
philosophers versus physicians, academics versus clinical professionals. For example, David Thomasma, a philosopher and early pioneer
in ethics consultations, argued that philosophers, once they have appropriate clinical experience, are best suited to offer insights and
methods of value discernments in clinical ethics consultations
(Thomasma 1991). Many took this to mean philosophers were better
trained in a more relevant field to do ethics than others, and ques-
tioned how nonphilosopher clinicians, and especially physicians,
could be objective observers in clinical ethical conflicts (Marsh 1992).
On the other hand, some, particularly physician ethics consultants,
have emphasized the role of clinicians in ethics consultation because
of their inherent grounding as clinical professionals, viewing the training in ethics consultation as a kind of subspecialty of clinical medicine
(La Puma and Schiedermayer 1994).

Such discussions and debates, though helpful in delineating the
pros and cons of various backgrounds, have also prompted turf battles. One way to overcome or avoid such battles is to define clinical
ethics consultation in terms that are both complete and minimal,
addressing the competencies that apply to the whole process of
ethics consultation, including the direct interaction with patients,
families, and clinical staff and the ethical analysis and consensus-
building toward a practical resolution. Such definitional recognition
demonstrates that expertise in ethics consultation is both practical

and theoretical, encompassing a broad range of applied skills acquired from clinical mentoring and experience as well as intellectual skills acquired from academic training. The intellectual skills include a basic understanding of ethical theories, principles, codes, and methods of case analysis, and a facility for logical analysis and reasoning (Jonsen et al. 2002). The applied skills revolve around basic clinical skills of communication and facilitation incumbent on any clinician to possess who works directly with patients toward practical clinical outcomes. These applied skills, which are necessary to facilitate desired ethical outcomes, are best learned through practice under expert supervision, as is the standard of training for most clinical caregivers. Just as those trained in academic fields like philosophical ethics are at an advantage regarding the academic, analytical skills, those who are trained healthcare workers, such as nurses and physicians, possess by virtue of their training and experience many of the clinical skills necessary for clinical ethics consultation. But it should be the aspiration of the beginning ethics consultant to be grounded in the relevant basic skill of both sides.

In 1998, a combined task force from the Society of Health and Human Values (SHHV) and Society for Bioethics Consultation (SBC), now the American Society for Bioethics and Humanities (ASBH), developed a comprehensive set of competencies for ethics consultation, titled *Core Competencies for Bioethics Consultation* (ASBH 1998). The report outlined a full range of knowledge and skills involved in ethics consultation. Recently updated, the core competencies are the only professionally sanctioned guidelines providing standards for determining competencies in ethics consultations. While professional controversy remains about the status of the core competencies within the profession of bioethics (primarily concerning whether such competencies should become the basis for professional certification), the report remains a helpful resource in making determinations about ethics consultation standards within an institution.

Simply put, individuals from a variety of backgrounds can be trained to become excellent ethics consultants. It has been our experience that skilled individuals from many academic and health-related fields have developed the necessary competencies, grounded both in clinical experience and an advanced understanding of clinical ethics, to do ethics consultations at a professional level. In the coming years, as ethics consultation becomes more professionalized, minimal qualifications, in terms of academic degrees and training, will have to be set. Ideally, we believe healthcare institutions should require that anyone who serves in the role of ethics consultant should have a minimum of a master's degree in bioethics or some advanced equivalent such as a one-year, full-time fellowship, along with a clinical degree such as an MD, MSN, MSW, or an academic degree such a PhD or JD degree. No doubt, having ethics consultants from a range of professional backgrounds is an advantage for the purpose of cross-disciplinary fertilization of ideas and perspectives.

THE NEED FOR A GENERAL APPROACH AND METHOD OF CASE ANALYSIS

Regardless of the professional background and training of the particular ethics consultant, a crucial question confronts anyone who might consider calling for an ethics consultation: what differentiates the input of the trained ethics consultant from an untrained, lay individual? Unlike most technical, scientific areas in which professional consultations are done in the medical setting, ethics is an area in which many people have an interest and legitimate stake and, often, strong opinions. It is the authors' view that what characterizes the approach of a qualified ethics consultant is the intelligent understanding and use of a method, which is the defined theoretical structure in which information (medical facts, value conflicts, ethical principles, and so forth) in ethics cases can be systematically gathered, analyzed, and resolved. So, properly used, a method provides assurance the ethics consultant has been fair-minded and thorough in executing a strategy and reaching a conclusion. To date, no one method for doing ethics consultation has been universally adopted, and as such, it may seem arbitrary to adopt any particular method. Before recommending a particular method we have found helpful, we believe there is a general approach that underlies most any method that requires the consultant's clinical involvement in the case.

There is widespread agreement that ethics facilitation is the most appropriate general approach for ethics consultations (ASBH 1998). Thus, as a general approach to doing ethics consultations, facilitation can be viewed as basic to a more specific method requiring the clinical involvement of the consultant. The primary characteristic of the facilitation approach is the open-ended way the ethics consultant approaches an ethics case with the attitude of assisting those involved in the conflict to arrive at an agreed-upon consensus. The facilitation approach is evident when the consultant makes his first encounter with the patient or family member central to a case. For example, a consult might start as follows:

> Hello, my name is [consultant's name]. I am an ethics consultant and have been asked by [whoever asked for the consult] to come and talk with you. I routinely get involved in cases where difficult ethical decisions must be made about the best course of action to take. I want to assure you that I do not have an agenda of my own with preconceived answers about what's right or wrong. My role is to talk with you and support you in considering the options that are available, and hopefully reach an outcome with which you are comfortable and that is in the best interests of your loved one. Is it ok if we talk?

Such an opening, which is the mark of facilitation, frames the consultant as someone there not to take sides with preconceived outcomes, but as someone who can listen, talk, and bring people together as much as possible in deciding what is best for the patient.

The facilitation approach in this chapter is viewed as the most general method of doing ethics consultations, compatible with more specific methods. It reflects the need to gather relevant information for the purposes of clarifying the nature of the value conflict so that the parties involved can be provided with an opportunity to come to a consensus within a structured, procedural process, consistent with well-established moral principles. The whole approach to facilitation assures, as much as possible, that the consultant's assistance toward any outcome is made on the basis of a fair and objective analysis of the value-laden expressions of beliefs and values, as well as the medical facts of the case. But for facilitation to be used, a more precise methodology of gathering and analyzing data and drawing conclusions must be adopted.

This chapter will use a model of ethics case analysis developed by Robert Orr and Wayne Shelton, based on their collaboration as clinical ethics consultants and educators. This model demonstrates how an ethics case can be fully analyzed and presented by a professional ethics consultant, and as such is both useful in practice and comprehensive in scope.

Table 4.1. Orr/Shelton: Format for Writing a Clinical Ethics Case Consultation Report

Step 1: Demographic data

Step 2: Reason for consultation request
Also, what is the key question that the requestor brought to the ethics consultant?

Step 3: Informants
Who were the individuals from whom you obtained information about the ethics consultation? They should be listed.

Step 4: Systematic Description of the Case
This section should be divided into four categories: medical indications, patient preferences, quality of life, and contextual features.

- Medical Indications—recent condition, baseline condition, current condition, treatment options, and prognosis.
- Patient Preferences—does the patient have capacity or not, stated wishes, advance directives, surrogates, and so forth.
- Quality of Life—baseline prior to current situation, current baseline, and probable baseline in the near and short term.
- Contextual Features—social and family situation, any other relevant factor such as religion, law, community values, caregiver bias, and so forth, that impinge upon this case, or on which this case impinges.

Step 5: Assessment
Based on the facts presented in the discussion, what is the basic condition of the patient and what is the basic ethical issue that arises?

Step 6: Discussion and Analysis
Based on your assessment, clarify, explore, explain, and analyze the key issues and conflicts in the case. Make sure you inform the reader of what is at stake in ethical terms (be sure to use ethical terminology such as rights, obligations, and values). Refer to relevant moral principles and clarify how they may be in conflict and argue how you think they should be prioritized. Also refer to any relevant precedent, particularly legal opinions, that may help to clarify your discussion.

Step 7: Recommendation
State succinctly the recommendations that follow from your discussion and analysis in a clear, precise, and practical way so as to elucidate the clinical caregivers' ethical obligations.

The Orr/Shelton model, though, was not developed in a vacuum, but instead draws from Jonsen, Siegler, and Windslade, in their book *Clinical Ethics* (Jonsen et al. 2002).

Orr/Shelton, however, provides a broader structure in which a factual and value clarification and analysis, value prioritization, and a precise recommendation can be made. We offer this method for the

Table 4.2. Jonsen et al.—The Four Boxes	
Medical Indications Consider each medical condition and its proposed treatment. Ask the following questions: • Does it fulfill any of the goals of medicine? With what likelihood? If not, is the proposed treatment futile?	*Patient Preferences* Address the following: • What does the patient want? • Does the patient have the capacity to decide? If not, who will decide for the patient? • Do the patient's wishes reflect a process that is informed? understood? voluntary?
Quality of Life Describe the patient's quality of life **in the patient's terms**: • What is the patient's subjective acceptance of likely quality of life? • What are the views of the care providers about the quality of life? • Is quality of life "less than minimal" (i.e., qualitative futility)?	*Contextual Features* Social, legal, economic, and institutional circumstances in the case that can: • influence the decision or • be influenced by the decision (e.g., inability to pay for treatment, inadequate social support)

beginning consultant to use to ensure thoroughness, but also for the seasoned consultant, particularly as a way of educating staff involved in the case how the original ethical conflict was understood, analyzed, and resolved. Below, then, is a description of the steps recommended.

—∞—

Step 1: Demographic Data

The first step is to ensure that important demographic information is being kept about the case. This information allows the ethics consultant to record, both for current and future use, crucial facts about the key participants, dates, and identifiers. Of course this is highly confidential information and must be kept in a safe and secure area but should be maintained as part of an ongoing database that will shed light on which units of the hospital ethics consultations originate from and the prevalence of certain kinds of issues that may need institutional attention. (Of course if any of these data are used in publishable studies, they must be de-identified, and Institutional Review Board approval must be obtained.)

Step 2: Reason for Consultation Request

Step 2 is usually the first information the ethics consultant is provided about the case. As the experienced ethics consultant knows, calls come from many sources and often when you least expect them. In most cases, the consultation begins with a request from someone actually involved in caring for the patient, usually a clinical caregiver, such as a nurse, resident, or an attending physician, but at times, the request may come from a family member of a patient, or even the patient him/herself. It is best to operate with the assumption that the person making the request presents information about the situation and their reasons for the consult request in good faith. At the same time, it is important to remember that the request comes from one of many perspectives. While there is no reason a priori for the ethics consultant to question the authenticity of this initial input of information, being a facilitator means first and foremost that information is to be gathered and acknowledged. The initially stated reason for the consultation provides a rationale or basis for launching the consultation process.

In a real sense, the initial reason, or preliminary ethical question, always requires further investigation by the ethics consultant, and that investigation can lead in one of three directions: First, the initial question may, once fully analyzed, prove the central and final question that actually warrants an answer. Second, fact gathering and analysis may require that the initial question be understood in a new way—that is, the initial question gets reframed, for example from a concern for principles to an issue of communication. And finally, though less frequently, investigation may determine that the initial question did not, in fact, pose an ethical conflict at all, in which case the preliminary ethics question is dissolved, for example, if it turns out to be just a misunderstanding.

Step 3: Informants

In the third step, the ethics consultant should record the informants in the case. "Informants" are the individuals with whom the ethics consultant had conversations and obtained information relevant to the case. In most cases, a key source of the nonmedical facts will come from the patient and/or the family, significant others, friends, or guardians. Talking to the clinical caregivers directly involved in the case is also important, both to clarify the medical facts and to get a richer overview of the case. Nurses, social workers, pastoral care givers, and other team members are often invaluable. The ethicist should be prepared to talk to any and all of these key players and to record what was reported.

Step 4: Systematic Description of the Case

Step 4 is the systematic description of the case. Here is the bulk of the work, since describing the case requires careful synthesis not only of given facts but expressed and operative values as well. This can be done in one of two ways: (a) a full descriptive narrative of the case, in all of its relevant medical and nonmedical aspects, can be provided, or (b) use of a more defined structure so as to ensure thoroughness is possible. The narrative approach is used by some experienced consultants as they are used to thinking through a case systematically, and a narrative account can tell a helpful story of how the ethical conflicts in a case emerged. The alternative, structured approach can be helpful especially for the beginning ethics consultant, though even the most seasoned consultant may find such structure useful. The structure recommended in this chapter follows closely the "four box" method of Jonsen et al. (2002; see Table 4.2).

Medical Indications

Once the initial reason for an ethics consultation has been determined, and the consultant makes her best effort to discern it, and accepts that it warrants an ethics consultation, the process begins; the essential starting place necessary to understand the value conflicts is with the medical facts of the case. The ethics consultant's role as a medical fact gatherer implies that he or she must be qualified to understand and assess medical facts at a basic level for the purposes of a nonmedical consultation, and must be able to function in the clinical setting as a trusted team colleague. Thus, the ethics consultant must be able to read through the patient's chart and, in discussion with medical staff, glean a clear and basic understanding of the medical facts, and will usually set the general physical parameters of the patient's condition and future decision-making goals.

One of the first questions the ethics consultant will ask is perhaps the most obvious: what is the patient's diagnosis and prognosis, and what are the viable medical goals of care for the patient, based on medical expertise? These are all factual questions based on medical evidence. It is important to note, "goals of care" should not be construed in any way as physicians' value-based preferences, but rather, an assessment of outcomes that are possible to be accomplished medically. Many other questions pertaining to the medical facts may need answers, such as: Can the patient survive with treatment? If so, will there be any disabilities or limitations? Is palliative care an option? What is the likelihood that the medical goals of care will be accomplished? Is there a reasonable likelihood, or are they impossible? All of this information must be expressed in ordinary nonmedical language, for the purpose of communicating to patients and families.

As the medical facts are gathered and analyzed, there often emerges a clearer perspective of the medical benefit-burden ratio. That is, how will the potential medical benefits that can or are likely to be accomplished for the patient, such as extended life, compare to the medical burdens, such as physical pain, suffering, and disabilities? This assessment is intended to be as value neutral as possible and should be based on an objective, scientific understanding of the case as reported by the attending physician and other expert clinicians involved in the case. The clearer the understanding of the benefit-burden ratio, the better able physicians are to fulfill their obligations to do good (beneficence) and not cause harm (nonmaleficence) to patients (Beauchamp and Childress 1994).

Patient Preferences

It could be argued that the ethics consultant enters the case to complement, and sometimes to repair, the physician-patient relationship by spending time listening and talking about the medical facts in relation to the patient's and family's wishes and values. The ethics-consultation process becomes an opportunity to clarify the goals of care from the patient's point of view, because the bedrock of contemporary medical ethics is respect for patient autonomy (that is, self-determination). Simply put, this means that the known wishes and preferences of patients should be heard and taken seriously as a guide to executing the medical care plan. There may be any number of reasons the patient and his surrogate(s) have that make certain medical goals more preferable than others. This principle of respect for patient autonomy applies to individuals who have or have had the capacity to express their values and preferences. This means that for young children (see chapter 9) and others who are not able, or who have never been able, to express their individual autonomy, the principle of respect for autonomy has no direct applicability. Rather, parents and guardians who are surrogate decision makers are viewed as having moral authority to be their decision makers, but must do so within the constraints of their best interests (PSDA 1990; Beauchamp and Walters 1999).

If the patient has capacity and is able to verbalize his or her wishes directly, then the ethics consultant should speak directly with the patient (Fletcher and Hoffman 1994). If the patient lacks capacity based on a thorough assessment (Buchanan 2004), the ethics consultant must attempt to discover the patient's prior wishes. Patients have the right to appoint a healthcare agent to make decisions for them and a right to have their prior expressed wishes honored, if they should be incapacitated (PSDA 1990). The person in the role of surrogate speaks on behalf of the incapacitated patient, and has the obligation to do so in a manner consistent with the patient's known values and preferences, as much as possible. However, most individuals do not appoint a formal healthcare agent, so when most patients lose capacity, it is often necessary to identify someone who knows the patient well and can speak on his or her behalf, for all intents and purposes with the same moral authority (although not always legal) as a formally appointed agent. Again, the key ethical role of a surrogate, whether formally appointed or not, is to represent the patient's values and preferences. If the patient's prior wishes are not known, then the surrogate should make decisions for the patient on the basis of best interests (Veatch 2003). Laws in the state in which the consultation occurs will regulate the legal authority of the surrogate to make decisions on behalf of the patient. The state law will apply not just to surrogates for adults who have lost capacity, but also for parents and guardians who are acting as decision makers for children and others without capacity (Beauchamp and Walters 1999).

Sometimes a brief conversation with the surrogate will lead to quick resolution, whereas other times, extended conversations will be necessary requiring a time commitment, which many physicians cannot or do not make. Extensive conversations with surrogates and families are particularly necessary if they have some personal or family stressor, such as lingering guilt or emotional stress, which becomes a barrier to medical decision making on the patient's behalf.

In those situations, the ethics consultant will attempt to bring the situation into focus and discuss it in relation to the patient's preferences and values. The goal is to listen and provide support to the surrogate, while facilitating greater clarity about the responsibilities of acting in that role.

Quality of Life

The rapid increase in the number of potentially therapeutic options available for patients in recent years not only means greater potential benefits for patients but also an increase in the potential for risks and burdens. In cases where the patient has capacity, the patient herself will almost always be given the opportunity to assess the benefit-burden ratio and make a judgment about quality of life that accords with her own values and preferences. The exception may be when the patient's decisions unreasonably impact others, for example an elderly capacitated patient who needs constant care wants to return home and be cared for by a disabled spouse. But where the patient lacks capacity, the surrogate, the care team, and others should try to assess the patient's current and projected quality of life in relation to her known values and preferences, based on any available advance directive. In the vast majority of cases, the patient's known prior preferences and values should guide decision making (although some have argued that the condition the patient is in, in fact, affects the person to such a degree that he or she may not be the same person; if true, this would invalidate the advance directive [Veatch 2003]).

Some of the most difficult cases ethically are those in which the patient is expressing a clear preference but capacity is extremely difficult to determine; one of the tasks of the ethics consultant in such cases is to provide an outside perspective. If the patient is expressing a strong preference, even when capacity is marginal or in question, the patient's voice should be acknowledged and considered as much as possible. From a practical point of view, if a patient with questionable capacity is strongly resisting a medical option intended to be beneficial, for example a nasogastric tube (for temporary nutritional support), toward an improved quality of life, the chances of its accomplishing a goal is reduced. Thus, practically speaking, the patient's willingness or ability to cooperate with the provision of any medical therapy, regardless of capacity, is a consideration that should be taken into account.

In cases where, after concerted clinical effort, the patient's values are determined to be unknown or unknowable, decisions should be made according to the best interest standard, as mentioned above, and take into account a broad range of perspectives, including legal. This is a controversial area of clinical ethics (Buchanan and Brock 1989), but there are a few basic points HEC members should keep in mind. If there is anyone, blood relative or otherwise, who knows the patient at all, such as an attendant at a nursing home, and they are willing to provide genuine input, their voice should be heard. To the extent a basis for patient autonomy is unavailable, decisions should be based on viable options that most reasonably promote humane medical goals and enhance the patient's quality of life. The ethics consultant should describe in detail the nature of any compromise that the patient will likely experience relative to his prior baseline level of function, and a thorough description of the potential burdens and benefits of all medical options. Some obvious compromises include imminent death, permanent loss of consciousness, impaired or altered mental state, and paralysis. It is important to keep in mind that assessing quality of life is inherently difficult, not in the least because of the inevitable element of uncertainty in the medical prognosis.

Contextual Features

This is the broadest area of fact gathering regarding any and all issues in the context case, from the micro to the macro setting, and is limited only by the ethicist's imagination. Often, particular cases are affected by factors outside the physician-patient relationship, for example contentious relationships among the care team, a difficult psychosocial situation, complex family issues, cultural and religious affiliations, legal and economic factors, and so on. Also, particular cases can affect other interests outside the case, such as the hospital's supply of blood or other scarce resources and its ability to help other patients in need of blood or types of limited care. Each case represents a unique configuration of contextual features, and it is up to the ethicist to delineate those that bear in a significant way upon the case, but also how the case bears on outside factors within the institution and the health system. Anything is possible from the dramatic to the mundane—from the impact of a potential lawsuit that is pending against the driver of an automobile who caused the accident responsible for the trauma that the patient suffered, to the cultural tradition of a family that refuses to disclose a terminal diagnosis to the patient, to the impact of giving blood transfusions to a dying patient on other patients with curable illnesses who may be denied that resource.

Step 5: Assessment

From the systematic description of the case provided by the four boxes, it is now possible to move onto Step 5 and make a brief assessment of the basic condition(s) of the patient and most basic ethical issue(s) in the case. This is the time to take notice of how the issue with which the consultation initiated is re-asked, reframed, or dissolved in light of what has been learned in the case. The assessment being made at this point is done on the basis of a best effort attempt to gather thoroughly the relevant information in the case. So this assessment is what could be called a considered and informed statement of the central issue or conflict, stated in the most succinct form.

Step 6: Discussion and Analysis

Now that the central issue is stated, a full discussion and analysis can take place in Step 6. The first task is to *clarify* the competing value claims, for example, between obligations and rights (physician's obligation to do good versus patient's right to act autonomously), between competing rights (physician's right to act according to conscience versus patient's right to act autonomously), and between competing moral understandings of what is right (family members whose beliefs differ about the goals of care). Clarification always means sustained reflection and discussion with colleagues concerning these competing claims. This may mean the need for more specific, focused conversations on key points, or conversation with and insights from specific case participants or colleagues with specialized knowledge or information. When as much clarity as possible is achieved, it is necessary to *prioritize* the competing value claims and to *justify* them based on well-established guidelines that must be applied to the case. For example, in a free society where patients who have capacity or whose wishes and values are fully known have prima facie moral authority, competing value positions can be analyzed and a determination made as to which position takes priority. Thus a key role of the consultant is to help assess the limits of patient autonomy in relation to other values and principles, such as beneficence, non-maleficence, and justice. But more often, the patient's known wishes or a prudential understanding of the patient's best interest will help to guide the case. The ethics consultant may have to advocate for and explain why one value position takes priority over others as one who is familiar with the procedural process that includes ethical theory, codes, principles, professional standards, and the law, and is able to discuss fluently the range of viable options with the parties in a case, and most importantly, to rule out ethically unacceptable options, such as ones that violate basic patient rights.

Step 7: Recommendation

Now the method of case analysis can be taken to its conclusion, Step 7, to recommend how best to proceed in the case. The recommendation will be based on the logical and practical flow of what has happened so far, reflecting an accepted consensus among the various parties involved. The recommendation should succinctly spell out what specific action to take. It should reflect the facilitation approach, which aims at a consensus of moral judgment and opinion about what is the most appropriate and beneficial outcome, given the facts of the case, and should be consistent with basic moral principles and the law. If ethics facilitation has not been able to reach a consensus of the parties in conflict, the consultant should seek input from others on the HEC and, based on their deliberation of the facts of the case and relevant ethical principles, lay out a carefully delimited range of all and only ethically permissible options. Also, it should be as specific and concrete as possible, clearly describing to clinical caregivers what actions they should take based on their ethical obligations. For example, if the conclusion is to respect the patient's right to refuse life-prolonging care, it will be necessary to spell out that this may mean making the patient DNR, discontinuing all interventions that are not intended for comfort, even blood draws, and making maximum comfort the goal of care even if it has the unintended side effect of decreasing respiration and increasing risk of death. This allows the practitioner to know what precisely to do in fulfilling his or her obligations to the patient, as illustrated in the following recommendations (see Table 4.3).

Two final points are worth emphasizing. The first is that the recommendation is not just the opinion or view of an individual ethics consultant. Rather, it should reflect the consensus that emerges from those involved in the case and whose views were part of the consultation process, including the HEC. And, second, although discussing cases in the abstract is a useful activity for gaining insight into clinical conflicts, viewing the case as an outsider is never the same as having direct experience and involvement in the case. Judgments about how competing value positions should be prioritized obviously are profoundly affected by the real relationships of those in conflict and the kind of consensus to which they come.

Table 4.3 demonstrates how to write up a case according the method just outlined, using the details of Case #1, in the final form as it might appear in a consultation report.

Table 4.3.   Case #1: Ethics Consultation Report

Step 1: Demographic data
Name of patient: Martha Doe
DOB 4-4-XX MR#: XXX1111000
Requestor: Dr. Smith, Resident
Attending Physician: Dr. Jones
Service: Hospitalist, Unit: A-5
Consultant: Ms. Consultant
Date: 10-10-03

Step 2: Reason for consultation request
Reason for consultation request, or the key question that the requestor brought to the ethics consultant?
What are the physicians' obligations to protect the patient in this situation?
How do we ensure that the patient has capacity and understands the risks of her decisions?

Step 3: Informants
Patient
Patient's brother
Resident
Nurse
Social Worker
Attending

Step 4: Systematic description of the case
Medical Indications
The patient is an eighty-six-year-old woman who fell from her wheelchair at her home on January 20, 1989, while experiencing dizziness and lightheadedness. She

was able to call EMS and was transported to the ED. Patient was found also to have a GI bleed. A colonoscopy was done and there were no serious findings. The GI bleed has resolved itself. Prior medical history includes hypertension and CHF (Congestive Heart Failure). Patient is currently stable and ready for discharge but is physically weak and would benefit from rehab first. At this point, for her to go back to her home and live alone, there is a serious risk of her falling again.

Patient Preferences
She is fully alert and oriented, although it is not easy to communicate with her due to her being hard of hearing. She is very adamant about her desire to go home, and expressed a strong fear of having to go to a nursing home. She is also refusing to go to a rehab facility, as she fears it would lead to her having to go to a nursing home. It would appear that she has capacity to make decisions for herself.

Quality of Life
Her quality of life prior to admission apparently had some limitations, for example she was in a wheelchair, but apparently she was able to function rather well and take care of her own needs, for example, go shopping with help, and pay her bills. However, her ability to be self-sufficient is probably waning. Although maintaining her independence would appear to greatly add to her quality of life, as she becomes more physically unable to care for herself in her own apartment, the increasing risk she poses to herself could also negatively affect her quality of life.

Contextual Feature
She has been living alone in an apartment prior to admission. She receives Meals on Wheels, and regular visits from a home health aid. Her closest relative seems to be her brother who is eighty-eight years old and lives in another state. I spoke to him by phone and he reported that he spoke with his sister yesterday and she sounded better than she did recently—in fact he reported that he thought she had capacity and she has always been obstinate. Regarding the issue of whether to let her return home alone, he said "let her try it" and "there's not much else to do" and "it's impossible to change her mind." There doesn't seem to be any other relatives who stay in close touch with her. She mentioned that she trusts the opinion of a local physician, who may be helpful in talking with her.

Step 5: Assessment
This patient is in frail health, and her fierce independence, which is admirable, poses a risk to her safety if her autonomy is respected and she returns home to live alone.

Step 6: Discussion and analysis
The physicians in this case rightly sense they have a beneficence-based obligation to protect an elderly patient in declining health, who is slowly losing her independence. It would appear to be correct that this patient poses a risk to herself if she returns home to continue living independently. At the same time, the patient is fully communicative and oriented and able to state her values and preferences, so her capacity appears to be intact. She insists on returning home and refuses to consider a

(continued)

Table 4.3.   (*continued*)

nursing home. Her brother confirms that she has always been very independent and that we should respect her wishes. Although the physicians' concern is fully warranted, a paternalistic intervention to disrespect this patient's preferences would not be justified. She has full capacity and her autonomy should be respected.

Step 7: Recommendation
Given that everyone seems to agree this patient has capacity, her right to have her wishes respected and followed should be honored. However, it is also true that her caregivers are correct to encourage her to consider rehab. In the end, her adamant refusal to follow her doctor's recommendations must override any obligation we have to protect her from herself, and she should be discharged according to her wishes.

METHODS OF RESOLVING CONFLICT

As should be evident from the description of the ethics consultation process in the above case, a key part of an ethics consultation is that it brings in a third party which engages in conflict resolution. HEC consultants must be able to use effective strategies that will help bring both sides closer to agreement. Traditionally, three roles have been defined for third-party conflict resolution in general: negotiation, arbitration, and mediation. Of these three roles, none captures completely what the HEC consultant does in the clinical setting, and confinement to one of these roles could possibly result in worsening the existing dilemma. As such, it will be useful to outline each of the three strategies and their application to ethics consultation; however, of the three, the role that is most often useful to ethics consultation is the role of the mediator, and its usefulness and significance has been developed in the literature (Bush 1989; Bush and Folgers 1994; Della Noce 2001; Moore 1996; Stulberg 1981; Dubler and Liebman 2004).

The purpose of negotiation is to bring the conflict to a conclusion that is favorable to the position of the party who requested the consultation. In general, this would be an inappropriate role for an HEC consultant since by definition, the consultation process is to be open-minded in order to collect evidence, listen to all sides, and build consensus. Thus, pure negotiation is probably the role that least captures what an ethics consultant does or should do. However, negotiation can be useful as a strategy if the terms of the options being negotiated have been established as ethically plausible, for example, in discussions with families who are making end-of-life decisions with physicians about when to withdraw artificial life supports for loved ones in multisystem organ failure. The ethics consultant, as well as other clinical caregivers, can negotiate a time frame with families who, although they understand the prognosis, are not ready emotionally to terminate treatment. The purpose is to agree upon a specific number of days in which to monitor clinical changes, before readdressing major decisions. Since there is no ethically predetermined time to withdraw treatment, and the only goal is to facilitate a decision consistent with the patient's best interests and family consent, a negotiated time frame can give the family a few extra days to prepare themselves for the patient's impending death, as well as a chance to accumulate additional evidence to confirm the prudence of the eventual decision.

Alternately, arbitration requires the consultant, at the request of both parties, to act as a judge. The arbitrator will start out gathering information from an impartial standpoint, but is expected to reach a conclusion at the end of the process. Both parties are bound to accept that conclusion. Rarely do ethics consultants have, or should they have, that kind of authority vested in them. Arbitration can, however, become part of the negotiation process, when a clinically skilled consultant facilitates a clinical dispute by acting as an arbitrator when both sides in conflict agree to recognize the consultant in that role.

Finally, the role of mediator is to help parties in conflict find and agree upon an acceptable solution. The mediator does this by providing a process for reaching a settlement, by asking and answering questions, clarifying answers, providing information, reframing difficult issues, and expressing empathy. The mediator does not take on the role of a judge but proceeds under the assumption that a common ground can always be found if there is enough facilitation of discussion and mutual understanding (Orr and deLeon 2000).

Nancy Dubler and Carol Liebman have developed useful guidelines for bioethics mediation in the clinical setting that include:

- Understanding the stated and latent interests of the participants
- Leveling the playing field to minimize disparities in power, knowledge, skill, and experience that separate the parties to the dispute

- Helping the parties define their interests, search for common ground, and maximize the options for conflict resolution
- Ensuring that the consensus can be justified as a "principled resolution," compatible with the principles of bioethics and legal rights of patients and families. (Dubler and Liebman 2004)

Following Dubler and Liebman's (2004) guidelines, the mediation process always starts out with an impartial stance regarding what should be the outcome of the case, and HECs must be given support from their institutions to maintain their stance (see chapter 15). The mediator's main focus is to maximize the likelihood of reaching a principled resolution by creating an atmosphere of neutrality where all the voices that have a stake in the outcome can be heard. In the example of negotiation of a time frame (above) we can imagine a different scenario where mediation would be appropriate—namely, if the physician failed to negotiate a time frame with the family and called an ethics consultant to resolve the impasse created by the disagreement about the appropriate time to withdraw treatment. In such a case, the goal of the ethics consultant would be to help the disputing parties through mediation to arrive at an acceptable time frame in which to make decisions about withdrawal of treatment.

MODELS FOR DOING ETHICS CONSULTATIONS

In addition to questions of expertise and qualifications, each institution that provides ethics consultation must consider what kind of model it wishes to use for providing this service. By "model," I mean institutional mechanism that defines what individuals will be responsible for providing the consultation, as opposed to "approach" and "method" used earlier, which have to do with the process in which it will be carried out. Of course, certain "models" accommodate, or not, certain "methods," as will become evident. The question of which model of consultation the HEC should adopt is often a matter of the kind of resources available, and HEC members should be able to assess within their institution what seems to be the best fit. There are three models for ethics consultations commonly used: (1) the individual consultant, (2) full committee, and (3) the small team.

The individual consultant is more common in large hospitals with frequent need for ethics consultations. No doubt, one of the key reasons this is so is that individual ethicists can move quickly to assist and make recommendations in cases that must be addressed urgently. They are on call and carry beepers like other clinical consultants and are able to respond to calls quickly. When a request for an ethics consultation is made, the individual consultant responds directly to the unit where the case is located to review the chart and converse with the participants. Often the issues can be resolved by consensus building reached through dialogue. However, in cases where the issues do not lend themselves to consensus, and especially where the case represents a deep conflict with legal ramifications, responsible ethicists should consult fellow ethicists, either in house or at other locations. The assumption is that no individual alone should be responsible unilaterally for making a recommendation about a deeply contentious value dilemma. Critical feedback from others is crucial to ensure that all sides have been examined and a reasonable recommendation is being made.

At the other extreme of the individual consultant model is the full committee. Because the HEC is made up of diverse individuals, it is hoped there are more points of view, and therefore a greater ability to analyze objectively the value conflicts that arise in ethics cases. Most of the members of an HEC are hospital staff with clinical orientations, such as physicians, nurses, and chaplains, and usually at least one community member. However, some HECs have a trained ethicist on board, but the level of ethics education of the members varies considerably. Often the members' education in clinical ethics is a result of informal programs developed by the HEC itself. Such self-education can be problematic since selection of educational material is being done by those who, themselves, may need education. Nevertheless, the advantage of using the full committee as a model for doing ethics consultations is that there are built-in checks and balances. Further, it provides for consideration of multiple perspectives brought forth by the members. Of course, there are downsides: first, since HECs are made up of a collection of individuals, it can be difficult to quickly mobilize a large group of professionals, getting them together in the same room. Second, it can be challenging to develop consensus about issues and getting them to agree on a recommended course of action (some other issues with committees are enumerated in chapter 15).

A compromise can be found in the small-team model, which usually consists of individuals from various professional backgrounds, such as nursing, medicine, pastoral care, and philosophy, appointed by the HEC because of their qualifications in the area of clinical ethics. Thus, this method retains from the committee method the inherent feature of multiple perspectives. This provides a built-in check process to ensure that delicate and controversial value-laden conflicts are managed as objectively as possible with no hint of a unilateral directive from one individual. And yet, unlike the full committee, because it is small, it can be quickly responsive to immediate situations. As Sulmasy points out, this approach has the advantage of "being rapidly responsive, clinically grounded and potentially very helpful to the healthcare team, patient and family. It also ensures that legitimate expertise will be present for the consult, because those who carry the beeper are expected to have met some standards of qualifications" (Sulmasy 2001, 101). Several other authors have recognized the advantages of the small-team approach, and it is becoming a common model of ethics consultation service within hospitals in the United States (Swenson and Miller 1992; Fox et al. 1998; Orr and deLeon 2000; Sulmasy 2001).

In the hospital in which Cases #1, #2, and #3 presented earlier took place, all began with an individual consultant responding to a call. However, in each case, the individual consultant sought advice and input from his fellow ethics consultants. In Cases #2 and #3 especially, it was necessary to involve a small team to discuss the issues and ensure thoroughness and objectivity. Both cases raised urgent and serious questions since they involved life-and-death decisions. The individual-consultant model allows a quick initial involvement and fact-finding in the case, but for cases like #2 and #3, a small team is optimal. The full committee may be useful at times, but only when there is ample time, which by the very nature of urgent difficult cases may not be typical.

CONCLUSION

This chapter has provided HEC members a basic overview of the ethics-consultation process in the hope of preparing them to fulfill their responsibility to oversee and perhaps participate in their ethics-consultation service. This overview has provided a sampling and description of typical ethics cases, the nature of the expertise required to consult, the steps in using a method to write up a case, the techniques used for conflict resolution, and the models of doing ethics consultations. We have learned in our own institution that an active HEC can create an atmosphere of interest in and increasing acceptance of ethics consultations. Our hope is that HEC members will use this basic information to promote the appropriate use of ethics consultations not only for the purpose of supporting their clinical staff, but also to increase the quality of care for patients and their families and friends.

Although the field of ethics consultation is developing rapidly, there is much work to be done in the future, and no doubt, HEC members will play a crucial role. There are many opportunities available for HEC members to learn more about ethics consultations from certificate programs, master's degrees, and fellowships in bioethics.

FOR FURTHER REFLECTION

1. What are the sources of ethical conflicts in the clinical setting?
2. How do ethics consultants help to resolve conflicts of value?
3. What counts as a "good" outcome?
4. What makes someone qualified to do ethics consultations?
5. Should there be professional standards to which ethics consultants are held accountable?

NOTE

The authors would like to acknowledge the excellent editorial assistance of Michelle Kilgallon in the preparation of this chapter.

WORKS CITED

ASBH. American Society for Bioethics and Humanities. 1998. *Core competencies for bioethics consultation*. Glenview, IL: American Society for Bioethics and Humanities.

Beauchamp, T., and J. Childress. 1994. *Principles of biomedical ethics*. Oxford: Oxford University Press.

Beachamp, T., and L. Walters, eds. 1999. *Contemporary issues in bioethics*. Washington, DC: Kennedy Institute of Ethics and Department of Philosophy, Georgetown University, Wadsworth Publishing.

Buchanan, A. 2004. Mental capacity, legal competence and consent to treatment. *Journal of the Royal Society of Medicine* 97:415–20.

Buchanan, A., and D. Brock. 1989. *Deciding for others: The ethics of surrogate decision making.* New York: Cambridge University Press.

Bush, R. A. B. 1989. Efficiency and protection, or empowerment and recognition? The mediator's role and ethical standards in mediation. *Florida Law Review* 41:253.

Bush, R. A. B., and J. P. Folgers. 1994. *The promise of mediation: Responding to conflict through empowerment and recognition.* San Francisco: Jossey-Bass.

Della Noce, D. J. 2001. Mediation as a transformative process. In *Designing mediation: Approaches to training and practice within a transformative framework,* ed. J. P. Folger and R. A. B. Bush, 71–84. New York: New York Institute for the Study of Conflict Transformation.

Dubler, N., and C. Liebman. 2004. *Bioethics mediation: A guide to shaping shared solutions.* New York: United Hospital Funds of New York.

Fletcher, J. C., and D. E. Hoffmann. 1994. Ethics committees: Time to experiment with standards. *Annals of Internal Medicine* 120 (4): 335–38.

Fox, M., et al. 1998. Paradigms for clinical ethics consultation practice. *Cambridge Quarterly of Healthcare Ethics* 7:308–14.

Hester, D. M. 2001. *Community as healing: Pragmatist ethics in medical encounter.* Lanham, MD: Rowman & Littlefield. Pp. 26–27.

Hollinger, P. C. 1989. Hospital ethics committees required by law in Maryland. *Hastings Center Report* 19 (1): 23–24.

Jonsen, A., et al. 2002. *Clinical ethics: A practical approach to ethical decisions in clinical medicine.* 5th ed. McGraw-Hill.

Kelly, D. F. 2004. *Contemporary Catholic health care ethics.* Washington, DC: Georgetown University Press.

La Puma, J., and Schiedermayer. 1994. *Ethics consultation: A practical guide.* Jones and Bartlett.

Lo, B. 1987. Behind closed doors: Problems and pitfalls of ethics committees. *New England Journal of Medicine* 317 (1): 46–50.

Marsh, F. H. 1992. Why physicians should not do ethics consults. *Theoretical Medicine* 13 (3): 285–92.

McGee, G., et al. 2001. A national study of ethics committees. *American Journal of Bioethics* 1 (4): 60–64.

Moore, C. W. 1996. *The mediation process: Practical strategies for resolving conflict.* 2nd ed. San Francisco: Jossey-Bass.

Noble, C. N. 1982. Ethics and experts. *Hastings Center Report* 12 (3): 7–9.

Orr, R., and D. deLeon. 2000. The role of the clinical ethicist in conflict resolution. *The Journal of Clinical Ethics* 11(1): 21–30.

PSDA. Patient Self-Determination Act of 1990. *Omnibus budget reconciliation act of 1990,* Pub. L. No. 101-508 4206,44751 (codified in sections of 42 U.S.C., in particular 1395cc, 1396a (West Supp. 1991).

Scofield, G. R. 1993. Ethics consultation: The least dangerous profession? *Cambridge Quarterly of Healthcare Ethics* 2 (4): 442–45.

Stulberg, J. 1981. The theory and practice of mediation: A reply to Professor Susskind. *Vermont Law Review* 6:85.

Sugarman, J. 1994. Should hospital ethics committees do research? *Journal of Clinical Ethics* 5 (2): 121–25.

Sulmasy, D. 2001. On the current state of clinical ethics. *Pain Medicine* 2 (2): 97–105.

Swenson, M. D., and R. B. Miller. 1992. Ethics case review in health care institutions; Committees, consultants, or teams? *Archives of Internal Medicine* 152 (4): 694–97.

Thomasma, D. C. 1991. Why philosophers should offer ethics consultations. *Theoretical Medicine and Bioethics* 12 (2): 129–40.

Veatch, R. M. 2003. *The basics of bioethics.* 2nd ed. Upper Saddle River, NJ: Prentice Hall.

Yoder, S. D. 1998. The nature of ethical expertise. *Hastings Center Report* 28 (6): 11–9.

5

Responsibility in Actual Practice

Consent and Participation in Clinical Ethics Consultation

Stuart G. Finder and Mark J. Bliton

KEY POINTS

1. Despite the fact that informed consent has been, and continues to be, a central ethical issue in health care, and, moreover, that the field of bioethics has been a major voice in promoting the need for informed consent in patient-care contexts, it is not automatically the case that patients or their surrogates must provide informed consent prior to the commencement of ethics consultation. The reason concerns both the general factor that clinical contexts are ethically complex and the more specific factor that, within any actual clinical circumstance, other participants in that circumstance may in fact carry a greater ethical burden and be subject to greater vulnerability than the patient.

2. When ethics consultation is understood as directed toward discovering and addressing the array of ethical considerations present in a given clinical circumstance, it follows that in any given clinical ethics consultation, it may or may not be appropriate to include patients, their surrogates, or their family members in the consultative process. Determining who ought to be included turns primarily on what is actually going on in the specific clinical circumstance and what is ethically at stake for the potential participants.

"Who ought to participate in an ethics consultation?" "Can ethics consultation be refused?" "Does there need to be consent before proceeding?" "If consent is necessary, from whom?" These are some of the more practical questions associated with responsibility and clinical ethics practice that are faced by those who serve on hospital ethics committees (HECs) and perform clinical ethics consultations. Unfortunately, there are no well-established answers to these questions, as they have seldom been directly and explicitly addressed in the academic bioethics literature. Instead, when it comes to the topic of responsibility and clinical ethics, attention has mostly been directed toward an array of more general considerations, such as the appropriate education and training of ethics consultants, the limits and scope of the ethics consultants' role; legitimate methods, formats, and objectives of ethics consultation; and how to conceptualize success, effectiveness, quality assurance, and other kinds of evaluative facets associated with ethics consultative practice. Not only that, but these considerations have primarily been addressed in academic, theoretical, or political terms, which often fail to appreciate that HEC ethics consultations occur in, and are focused on situations which arise out of, a "clinical" context. And the fact that ethics consultations are *clinical* is significant.

First, clinical circumstances are composed of unique sets of interpersonal relationships—between this patient and these care providers, this patient and her family, this family and those care providers, among these care providers themselves, and so on. Such relationships are further influenced by more general facets of professional and institutional considerations, which are themselves shaped by and reflective of economic, political, religious, and other perspectives, histories, norms, commitments, and so on. Accordingly, in actual clinical circumstances, the relational dynamics among the various participants are neither singularly unique nor fully general (Zaner 1993).

In addition, the clinical context is one in which continual change (Cassell 1991), inherent uncertainty (Pellegrino 1983), and dependence upon unavoidable and complex forms of trust (often among relative strangers) (Zaner 1988) pervades the routines, expectations, and experiences of all those who must choose and act within such contexts. Accordingly, the meanings of each clinical choice and decision, and subsequent actions, are deeply embedded within complex and dynamic webs of cultural and social relationships among just those individuals participating in the specific circumstance (Bliton and Finder 1999).

Furthermore, and perhaps more dramatically, the dynamics that characterize clinical contexts are bound by time. But this is not the time of well-crafted stories in which events and decisions are stitched together by a definitive narrative thread. Certainly, like good stories, clinical events have clearly demarcated beginnings and, eventually, identifiable ends, and the events and decisions that link beginning to end may be retrospectively seen as having done so in their own specified time. However, as encountered in the midst of actual clinical circumstances, time is not experienced as predetermined and necessarily leading to this or that specific end. Rather, it is unfolding, and the press of this unfolding time is often urgent. Moreover, the many participants in the specific clinical circumstance are, so to speak, acting in an ongoing present. What connects this present with the continually reevaluated past, furthermore, are the choices actually chosen, the decisions actually decided, the actions actually enacted. Clinical contexts, in other words, are never passive, never still; they are active. As such, *clinical* significance places a premium on that which is actualizable—that is, the specifically practical. In this sense, theory and abstraction have little place—except insofar as they might serve to guide or direct action in general (on the way to the particular).

While it is likely that any ethical view we hold may make demands on our lives, our actions, and our other commitments, the task of *clinical* ethics consultation, then, is one of looking into a situation, in all its rich detail, in order to figure out what is specifically at issue—and why—and then what can be done about it, all without compromising the evident commitments held by those individuals in that situation. Moreover, that kind of discovery and clarification needs to be accomplished by interacting with the people whose situation it is, for it is precisely *they* who face making decisions and who must then live in the aftermath of whatever decisions are eventually enacted (Zaner 1988). Therefore, independent of how the more general debates centered around responsibility are resolved within the field of bioethics more broadly, what matters for practitioners of clinical ethics consultation is that they must be attentive to the significance and shifts among context-dependent meanings, and the relational dynamics that shape such meanings (Bliton and Finder 2002).

In view of the above, we maintain that to identify and clarify the most morally relevant issues for a given clinical situation, and thus as an important step toward being responsible, individuals who serve as clinical ethics consultants or as members of HECs need a careful and deliberative process that can accommodate the varied and sundry forces associated with clinical contexts. It is our contention that actual ethics consultation thus requires careful questioning (regarding the complicating factors in the situation) and attentive listening (to the answers given), all the while seeking to make explicit what may be otherwise implicit. That kind of focus itself helps to situate one of the questions with which this chapter is concerned: "Who ought to participate in an ethics consultation?"

In raising that question, we do not intend to discuss the qualifications, training, expertise, and so on of those individuals who serve in the role of ethics consultants or as members of HECs. Instead, focus is on all those others who may potentially be included in the activities of ethics consultation via interaction with ethics consultants and HECs: patients and families, attending and other physicians, nurses, therapists, technicians, and so on.[1] There is practical import to determining who ought to participate. As we discuss in this chapter, the answer to this question cannot be divorced from the substantive ethical features of the specific circumstance in which clinical ethics consultation occurs.

To illustrate the moral grip of this initial question, we must focus as well on another question: Is informed consent for ethics consultation necessary? As it turns out, this question has received scant attention within the clinical ethics literature (Veatch 2001). When it has been addressed, the conclusion has been almost without exception the same— consent is required (Veatch 1989; Wolf 1991; Fletcher 1992; Arnold 1994; Roberts et al. 1995). We challenge that conclusion in this chapter as a way of showing that the question itself can be of great practical importance for the actual engagement in clinical ethics consultation.

SETTING THE CONTEXT: FOUR SCENARIOS

Brief Caveat and Clarification

Below are four scenarios. Their primary purpose is to exemplify the arguments and points concerning consent and participation in the context of ethics consultation, which are presented in this chapter.

The four scenarios are not, however, random examples. Rather, they represent three basic categories (the first two scenarios represent crucial variations of the first category) of the more common kinds of concerns those who perform clinical ethics consultations are likely to encounter. These categories are presented not as definitive frames into which all consultative instances will neatly fit, but merely as useful heuristic devices.

That being said, we are also aware that what counts as, and is meant by, "clinical ethics consultation" has been conceptualized in a variety of ways, not all of which are compatible (Aulisio et al. 1999). However, there is little debate that end-of-life situations serve as a kind of paradigmatic example for many both within the healthcare professions and the lay community. Accordingly, the scenarios we offer address situations revolving around end-of-life decision making.

1. Interpersonal Relational Dynamics: Patient/Family–Physician

Several days ago, after a prolonged course of chemotherapy (most recently under an investigational protocol) for a primary lung cancer that has metastasized to the pelvis and spine, Dr. Tom McMillan, the oncologist in charge of Janice Pear's care, told her family that there were no more options available, that she would not survive to see her fifty-third birthday next month. In fact, Dr. McMillan told them it was most likely she would not live through another week. Her husband, James, and their two children, Larry, 28, and Ken, 25, who have actively participated in her care throughout her long course, and whose commitment and devotion to her has been praised by both the medical and nursing staffs, were deeply saddened by this news. But, they admitted that they were not surprised.

Appreciating how difficult it can be for families to absorb such news, Dr. McMillan arranged for another meeting with the family for the following day. During that meeting, attended by Dr. McMillan, Dr. Richard Worthington, the ICU attending physician, Megan Johnson, one of the charge nurses, and Mrs. Pear's family, it was agreed that from this point forward, the emphasis of care would shift from curative to palliative, with the goal of keeping Mrs. Pear as comfortable as possible as she dies. After the meeting, Megan stayed with the Pear family in the meeting room to answer any additional questions they might have about what would happen and to provide additional emotional support.

It was thus a surprise early this morning, right after shift change, when James Pear approached Megan and angrily accused the just-departed night nurse of administering too much narcotic for his wife. Moreover, he alleged that the nurses were trying to hasten her death now that the physicians have stated that she will not recover. He demanded to speak to someone in the hospital about what he takes to be a serious breach of ethics.

Megan, in a manner that her nurse colleagues deeply respect and for which she is well-regarded among the ICU physicians, told Mr. Pear that she could readily understand his frustration over what was going on with his wife, and that she would certainly pass his concern along. Unfortunately, Mr. Pear interpreted her response as an effort to diminish his concern since, as he said to her, "This is not about frustration on *my* part, it's about *you and your nurses* trying to kill my wife!" He continued, "I thought you, of all people, understood that my Janice is a fighter. But you're just like all the rest of them!" And then he stormed out of the unit.

Although a bit shaken, Megan did not take this personally; she believed Mr. Pear's outburst was nothing but an expression of his undergoing the experience of his wife's dying. She nonetheless also believed it important to pass his concern along through the proper channels. Accordingly, she immediately called and left a message requesting ethics consultation. She also told Dr. Worthington, when he came onto the unit a little bit later, about the situation and her request. After making sure she was OK, he told her he agreed with her action. He did, however, express concern when hearing that she had yet to speak with Dr. McMillan. As he said, "Mrs. Pear is Dr. McMillan's patient and he, not the ICU team, has ultimate responsibility regarding what is to be done."

2. Interpersonal Relational Dynamic: Intrafamily

A little over three years ago, when he turned eighty-five years old, Billy Freeman told his physician of seventeen years that if and when the time came that Billy could no longer make decisions for himself, and his physician believed there was little hope that medical interventions would be helpful, Billy did not want aggressive treatments nor did he want to be placed in a nursing home. Instead, he wanted to be cared for by his children. Mr. Freeman had actually gone to the effort of having a lawyer spell this out in a document, which he then had all five of his children sign as both an acknowledgment of their agreement with this plan and as a pledge to carry out his wishes.

Now, at eighty-eight years of age, Mr. Freeman's ability to care for himself was limited. His body and vitality were withered from a combination of advancing age and numerous ailments, including diabetes, renal failure, congestive heart failure, COPD, rheumatoid arthritis, near blindness, and near deafness. His mental faculties were also in decline due to a slow but steady worsening dementia. For the past six months, he had been in and out of the hospital five times, and despite aggressive medical interventions each time, his overall condition was declining. Most recently he had been admitted with his third bout of pneumonia for the year, in congestive heart failure, acute renal failure, and mental decline. He now was stable and ready for discharge. Mr. Freeman's physician felt the time had come: Mr. Freeman would not go home, but should instead spend his remaining days in the care of his family.

Unfortunately, there is a problem. Mr. Freeman's oldest child, Joanne, is domineering and, having spent all of her time at the hospital trying to micromanage the nurses, Mr. Freeman's physician, and anyone else involved in Mr. Freeman's care, she now insists Mr. Freeman go home with her and her husband Frank. Rene, the middle of the five children, believes Joanne, given her personality and the kind of care Mr. Freeman would need at this point, is ill-equipped to take care of him. She instead thinks Mr. Freeman should go to her older brother Billy Jr.'s home, which, she has argued, is more centrally located than either her own or Joanne's, plus Billy Jr. has greater economic resources than either of them. Billy Jr., as it likely has always been, is not so sure he wants to get on his older sister's bad side and hence has yet to commit either way. Kelly, the youngest daughter and the fourth child, has said that she's well accustomed to these sorts of disputes among her siblings and so is more than happy to have the others figure it out. And finally, there was the youngest child, Tim who, despite being fifty years old, is still referred to by his siblings as "Timmy" because he is nearly eight years younger than Kelly and sixteen years younger than Joanne. During the illness and dying of their mother, and then again for the dying of their father's second wife, Tim had been most involved in helping Mr. Freeman, and hence he believes he is best disposed to take care of his father now. But, as it has likely been in many of the moments of their lives as a family, he is still "little Timmy" and his oldest three siblings are all in agreement that he, at least, should be dismissed as the possible caregiver.

In view of all of this, Mr. Freeman's physician has had the bedside nurse call the HEC and ask for some help figuring out what to do.

3. Institutional Considerations: Policies,
Guidelines, Regulations, and Laws

Rachel Williams is a seventeen-year-old young woman who, twelve weeks ago, was diagnosed with an ostesarcoma believed to be responsive to a common chemotherapeutic regimen. She thus began chemotherapy eight weeks ago and has, to date, completed two rounds; she was scheduled to begin another round this week. However, due to ongoing and worsening complications related to her treatment—including the recent development of a bright erythematous rash, mucositis, intermittent nosebleeds, mild diarrhea, and fever—she is now hospitalized.

While none of this is desirable, it is not unexpected; these are common side effects of the regimen Rachel is receiving, and with appropriate intervention, it is expected that she can get through this temporary "bump" in her road to recovery. However, Dr. Jan Roberts, who is Rachel's oncologist, is concerned. The reason is that Rachel and her mother (her parents are divorced and her father lives out of state) are Jehovah's Witnesses, and during one of their first meetings with Dr. Roberts, Rachel's mother clearly stated that Rachel is not to receive blood transfusions. When this conversation occurred, Rachel too stated that she did not want to be transfused and that she understood that should a life-or-death situation arise in which her physical life could be saved by transfusion, she would still choose to refuse blood since to accept it would condemn her soul to eternal damnation. She also stated that now that she has become a full-fledged member of the church, she does not see this as a choice even her mother could overrule.

At this point, transfusion is not an immediate issue, although Rachel's hematocrit is down and her white blood cell count is elevated. Dr. Roberts can anticipate that should Rachel's condition deteriorate, the issue of transfusion may become crucial. She knows from past situations involving children who are Jehovah's Witnesses that she can ask for a court order so as to obtain the legal authority to provide blood if needed. However, she is unsure if, once she requests a court order, whether she is then obligated to provide transfusions. Moreover, since it is no secret that Rachel is a Jehovah's Witness, Dr. Roberts is a bit concerned that even if she gets a court order, there may be colleagues—both medical and nursing—who would not be supportive of forcing Rachel to undergo transfusion.

It is due to these circumstances that Dr. Roberts has asked the HEC for an ethics consultation.

4. Moral Disruption: Caring for Another, Deciding and Choosing, Living in the Aftermath

Stan Carmichel was admitted nearly two weeks ago to the burn unit after being in a house fire. The worst of his injuries were the extensive burns to his hands and forearms, undoubtedly caused as he tried to shield himself when the ceiling fell in. This also accounts for why the burns to his face are not nearly as bad as they could have been, although he did suffer serious injury to his eyes.

It was the inhalation injury, though, that had Stan's physicians most concerned. Hands are hard to heal without ending up with some sort of contractures, but with good rehab, Stan could certainly be able to regain the skills needed for some basic self-care, and even if he lost his eyesight, the facial burns should be able to be successfully grafted. But lungs are another story, and like many burn victims, Stan's pulmonary condition had quickly deteriorated while still in the ED, and around day five or so, shifted into ARDS.

Despite all of this, his burn physician has maintained optimism. She has certainly seen patients with much more extensive burns (despite the initial claim by the paramedics that his burns were 60 percent of his total body surface area [TBSA], it is now felt that Stan suffered only a 25-percent TBSA burn), and the extent of lung injury is notoriously difficult to predict. In fact, for as poorly as Stan's pulmonary function was doing as he concluded his first week in the hospital, his burn physician was anticipating that he'd likely be ready for extubation in an additional four to six weeks (assuming he continued on his current trajectory), could possibly leave the ICU two weeks after that, and be discharged to rehab after another two weeks, making his hospitalization only ten weeks.

The medical and nursing staff in the ICU were thus taken aback when, on day eight, Stan's three brothers requested that life support be withdrawn and Stan be allowed to die. In view of this, the ICU attending physician, Stan's individual burn attending physician, and the chaplain each met separately with Stan's family to learn more about why they were making this request at this time. And, all three had come to learn the same thing: although Stan had been serving as a "care partner" for the gentleman who had died in the fire, Stan had actually not been required to do much, that he was more a friendly companion than a valet for the man, and contrary to the image of him his physicians and nurses had created, Stan not only suffered from severe anxiety and depression, but in high school, he had been diagnosed with a borderline IQ. The man for whom he worked was a very close church friend of Stan's parents, and after his wife died ten or so years ago, he offered to take Stan in, provide room and board, in exchange for having Stan help him around his house. It was just the right kind of structured environment that his parents had hoped he'd find since, as they were getting older, they were starting to worry about what would happened to Stan once they died.

Stan's brothers also told how two years ago, after Stan's parents had both died very closely together (his mother from breast cancer, his dad, two months later from a massive MI), the brothers had, in fact, taken up the role their parents had been providing Stan, taking turns visiting him three to four times per week, to help him with whatever chores with which he might need help, and simply to visit. Even so, with his parents both gone, Stan had gone into a depression which took several months to clear. Continuing the kindness that he'd already shown in taking Stan in, the man for whom Stan worked allowed him to remain in his home during these months, and all agreed that, in the end, this had probably done more to help Stan than anything. Stan still suffered occasional bouts of depression in relation to his parents' passing, but the regularity of his schedule with this friend of his parents allowed him to get through them.

But now this man too was dead, and the brothers feared that this loss itself, should Stan recover, would be devastating. They also worried that Stan's being significantly debilitated—unable to use his hands, blind, with compromised and limited lung capacity—would only make matters worse for him. Plus, they understood that if Stan survived the current hospitalization, he'd need not just the obvious rehabilitation, but likely many return visits to the plastic surgeon for grafting, revascularization, and so on. Given all that they'd seen him go through, and knowing how he had responded to his life so far,

Stan's brothers did not believe Stan would be able to withstand this—emotionally, psychologically, spiritually. And so they had made their request. They stated, moreover, that they were in the best position to know Stan and how he would respond, that they knew his values and his beliefs, and that Stan would not want to undergo the kind of suffering that was inevitable both for his current care and for any future care should he survive.

The chaplain and the ICU attending felt that Stan's brothers were genuinely concerned for his welfare, that there were no hidden agendas or secondary gains, and that, if what they told of Stan's life was accurate, then there was merit to the brothers' request. Stan's primary burn physician, however, was unsure. She understood Stan's brothers' perspective, could even sympathize with it. But she couldn't shake that question of whether she would be doing the right thing if she agreed to stop everything now. For several days, she had been reviewing the arguments and rehearsing the possible justifications on both sides, of why it would be appropriate to stop, and why continuing to push forward could be justified. But she remained torn. Even when Stan's pulmonary condition deteriorated and he required greater ventilatory support just to keep his saturations in the upper eighties, his burn physician couldn't shake the feeling that backing off on Stan's interventions might not be the right thing to do.

Now, on the thirteenth day of Stan's hospitalization, his burn physician requests an ethics consultation.

IS CONSENT REQUIRED FOR CLINICAL ETHICS CONSULTATION?

The first question we take up is that of consent in the context of clinical ethics consultation. While the term (if not also the core concept of) "informed consent" originated within the U.S. legal context (Faden and Beauchamp 1986), the concern for informed consent has been, and continues to serve as, one of the touchstone considerations in bioethics. The reason is that informed consent is ultimately concerned with the question of responsibility, especially in light of the recognition that patients, due to illness or injury and the need for help, are, in many fundamental ways, significantly dependent upon physicians, nurses, and health care institutions for their care. Being vulnerable as such, patients are susceptible to exploitation—even if unintended. How best to respect patients and limit their vulnerabilities is thus a crucial, ethical question. And indeed, practical concerns about respecting patient preferences, limiting patient vulnerability, and avoiding potential exploitation often serve as the prompt for requesting ethics consultation.

Thus, it may seem striking, if not ironic, that the question of whether patients and their surrogates should be able to refuse clinical ethics consultation—or, at the very least, whether they must be notified before an ethics consultation may proceed—has received so little attention within the bioethics literature. It may also be notable that few authors have attempted to argue that the answer to such a question might be "no" (Bemis 1994; Finder 1995). Perhaps equally striking is that some within bioethics have seemingly assumed—if not outright asserted—that *attending physicians needed to give permission* before an ethics consultation can proceed for one of their patients (Purtilo 1984; Perkins and Saathoff 1988; LaPuma et al. 1992; Simpson 1992).[2]

What is most striking, however, is that the issue of patient refusal or physician permission assigns prominence and priority to an individual (patient or physician) based on that individual's *role* as opposed to what may be, or actually is, at stake for that individual in that situation. As such, *whoever* it is that occupies the role is taken as having *the most important stake* in what is raised. Presupposed, then, is that the patient or physician, or both, are empowered by their *role* to determine how others, in *their* roles, are not merely to act, but are also to understand and experience the situation.[3]

The problematic associated with this prioritization of role is particularly pronounced when considering those situations in which the "moral experience" of a care provider is at issue, such as in the fourth scenario. In that situation, it is very difficult to imagine what sort of rationale would conclude that it is legitimate for Stan Carmichel's family to prevent the HEC from trying to help Stan's physician as she struggles with her own moral understanding of the choices which confront her. Granting them that authority, in fact, undercuts the very notion of the need for a relative balance of power within patient–care provider relationships in order to limit patient vulnerability and potential exploitation—which is itself a core basis for informed consent—and the subsequent stance that patients cannot be forced by physicians, nurses, and so forth, to undergo interventions (a similar argument is used to counter the claim that physicians must give permission for ethics consultation; see Wolf 1991; Fletcher 1992).

More to the point, in any actual clinical circumstance, whatever is at stake for each individual are matters (that is, activities, experiences, information, understandings, and so on) for which that individual's role clearly serves as the access point by which that individual now is within the specific situation. In addition, the individual's role may also limit and shape how that individual experiences, understands, and makes sense of what is occurring both to oneself and to the others with whom one interacts. *But*, "what matters," that is, what is at stake for each individual, concerns more fundamental existential and moral facets connected to the individual's moral identity and self-understanding, including the extent to which one's commitments reach the depth of one's concern for this or that knowledge, relationship, value, and so on.

In the case of Stan's burn physician, as she contemplates her choices, she may likely take into consideration such matters as professional standards, practice guidelines, and so on, all of which are focused on the role of "physician." But in the end, it is she who must act—in the role, to be sure, but not solely so, given that the moral implications, for both herself and others, exceed what is established by those professional standards, practice guidelines, and so on. As such, she is not concerned with what *any physician* should do; she is trying to figure out what *she should do* and *how she will do it in this very situation*. The point, then, is this: it is not the role of "patient" or "physician" alone that serves as the primary basis for one's accepting or rejecting that attention be directed to ethical considerations; there is something quite significant about the individual who occupies a role.

That raises a crucial and more fundamental issue: if an ethics consultation will turn attention toward an individual's moral experience (as in the fourth scenario), or broad ethical frameworks within which patient care takes place (as in the third scenario), or the ethical dimensions of that individual's relationships within the specific clinical context (as in each of the first two scenarios), can that individual explicitly refuse such attention? Here the problem is more complex, for several reasons.

First, and possibly foremost, the reason that prompts a request for ethics consultation is not always identical with what turns out to be the most pressing ethical consideration in the situation. At the beginning of any ethics consultation, any attempt to conclude just who it is from whom consent must be sought is likely to be premature (unless the premise that patients must always give consent is simply asserted and the practical moral considerations raised earlier in this chapter are ignored). Second, if the ethical considerations are of the kind presented in the first two scenarios (that is, primarily concerned with interpersonal relational dynamics), then efforts are not directed to just one individual as if in isolation from consideration of the others also participating in that clinical situation. When the issues are relational, in other words, no *one* individual has ultimate say. Nevertheless, what if one of the individuals refuses while another agrees? Can the one who refused to participate in ethics consultation be compelled to participate?

Precisely here the issue of complexity in clinical situations, of itself, must become a primary consideration, because on the one hand, while the one who refuses ethics consultation cannot be given the power to prevent directing attention to the concerns and issues of another who agrees, so too is it the case that simply because one agrees does not indicate that the other who refuses is now required to have to participate in the ethics consultation. And so, when the issues identified in ethics consultations arise in and are focused upon the relational dynamics, it is reasonable that individuals may refuse to participate. However, the point is that their refusal cannot extend beyond their own participation; the process of ethics consultation may still move forward.

One further necessary clarification is needed regarding these issues. Since the request for ethics consultation comes to the HEC by an individual directly involved in the situation, on the basis of that request, the HEC is warranted to begin its process of discovering what is going on with the individual and in the situation that prompted the request. As such, the request itself serves as a kind of consent, from the requestor at least. As for the others involved in the situation, there is a difference between all those who, like members of the HEC, are part of the institution, and those (patients, families, and so forth) who are not. The reason is that there are in institutional life many different kinds of presumptions that allow the diverse individuals who constitute the institution to function with some degree of unity. Part of this is the idea—enacted daily via the variety of tasks and activities each member of the institution performs—of presumed mutuality of purpose and a sense of shared aims such that all within the institution are said to be, in a variety of ways, "colleagues." At least to this extent, there is a kind of presumed consent built into the system during the early stages of discovering what is going on insofar as colleagues qua colleagues place trust in each other and grant provisional latitude while involved in determining what one should do.

The same, however, cannot be said for the patients and families who do not "belong" to the institution. Even though trust is inherent to the relationship between patient and physician, patient and nurse, and so on, and even if a patient regularly receives care in this particular hospital, patients are not members of the institution. Indeed, no matter how regularly patients and families interact with the institution, each clinical encounter requires a renewed focus, and as such, they cannot be presumed to agree; they must be asked.

In summary, it is important to note that these complexities of the first category of ethics consultation—those focused on interpersonal dynamics—highlight a theme crucial to moral experience, namely, that moral experience is not solely defined or regulated by the role one occupies in a particular situation. Hence, in the first scenario, Dr. Worthington's concern about Megan's experience is legitimate and is not constrained by the authority of Dr. McMillan (whereas other aspects of the ICU team's involvement in the situation may be so constrained). Similarly, any number of individuals in a specific situation (including physicians and nurses) may be legitimately concerned about suffering (a preeminent moral consideration) even though such concern does not fall under the purview of any one or another professional discipline. Thus, ethics consultants and members of HECs who encounter these kinds of matters are well advised to pay careful and specific attention to what is actually going on in the particular circumstance.

What about those ethics consultations that are focused on institutional considerations, as in the third scenario above: does it make sense to say that Rachel or her parents need to be asked in order for the HEC to address Dr. Roberts's concern? Dr. Roberts wants to know more about court orders and is looking for advice about how to manage possible disagreements or disruptions from fellow staff (medical and nursing). Were the context changed only slightly, for instance, if Rachel was a Jehovah's Witness refusing transfusion and facing the possibility of surgical intervention, and instead of court orders, Dr. Roberts wanted to know more about the ramifications of attempting bloodless surgery, or even more specifically, different techniques for limiting blood loss (as well as advice regarding subsequent interactions with the staff), would it make sense to ask Rachel or her parents for consent before Dr. Roberts could inquire about those issues? It is difficult to imagine that the question of Rachel's or her parent's consent would be raised even though what Dr. Roberts finds out might make a difference in terms of the options she presents to Rachel and thus how she proceeds in her care of Rachel. The issue at stake, in other words, is that the prompt for Dr. Roberts's concern and eventual request for ethics consultation is not only focused on Rachel per se. Although motivated by Rachel's being a Jehovah's Witness and adamantly stating she does not want to be transfused, in a significant sense, Dr. Roberts's inquiry is not limited to Rachel's situation. Dr. Roberts's inquiry is about a specific category into which Rachel and her situation may be placed: juvenile Jehovah's Witness refusing blood products for whom blood products may have some physiological benefit. And here, then, is the crux: the specific circumstances point toward something more general, and thus become the occasion to explore that more general concern. In that light, the question of informed consent simply doesn't fit; it's a non-issue at this time.

Returning to the ethics consultations focused on the moral experience of the requestor, connections with all that has been discussed so far may be traced. For instance, it may be useful for the HEC to meet with Stan Carmichel's brothers in order to appreciate the kind of experience the burn attending physician is having. But is such a meeting necessary? No. It may be more to the point to meet with this physician and allow her time to discuss and work her way through that which she is experiencing. Accordingly, akin to some ethics consultations that revolve around relational dynamics, it may be useful to involve Stan's family, and if so, they should be asked if they are willing to participate in meeting with the HEC. Their answer, however, does not present a limit to keep the HEC from proceeding in discussion with the burn physician. Similar to what was suggested above, just as moral experience is not to be understood as falling under the purview of any one professional discipline or institutional role, so too is it the case that any one individual occupying a role or fulfilling a professional discipline cannot dictate whether the moral experience of any other individual in the situation is to be addressed.

As mentioned at the beginning of this section, the issue of informed consent is often seen as a touchstone consideration within bioethics, and its context is clearly clinical. What has been discussed above is meant to demonstrate, however, that even though it is a crucial issue for the field, within the actual context of a specific clinical ethics consultation, informed consent may or may not be fitting. The determinants will be the actual circumstances of the situation. Accordingly, maintaining a policy or protocol that requires that informed consent be obtained prior to pursuing a clinical ethics consultation may betray the very clinical elements that define that particular situation and give rise to those issues for which ethics consultation has been sought.

PROMOTING PARTICIPATION: IS MORE BETTER?

The question of who ought to be included in the various activities associated with ethics consultation, and thus participate with ethics consultants and HECs in clinical ethics interactions, has received virtually no attention in the clinical ethics literature since the mid-1990s. Why is that? Some have suggested this is the result of wide cultural and social acceptance of clinical ethics consultation as a legitimate practice. As such, matters such as clinical ethics methodology, composition of ethics consultation teams, quality assurance and evaluation, and documentation of process have greater priority in order to satisfy the practical and political needs of actual HECs and clinical ethics consultation services (Rubin and Zoloth-Dorfman 1994). The question of who ought to participate, in other words, has been shunted aside by more pressing concerns.

This question may also have lost its poignancy due to the fact that the legalistic notion of self-determination, stressing as it does the primacy of autonomy, has often been taken as central to the venture of clinical ethics (Agich and Youngner 1991). Accordingly, processes that do not allow the patient (if capable) or the patient's representative (when the patient was incapable) to participate have been taken to be in opposition of the accepted need to respect patient autonomy.

Whether either of these accounts is accurate, it is clear that the question regarding participation has been seen as settled for some time. Over the years, it has simply warranted no further attention. However, maintaining the stance that this question is no longer relevant fails to account for what is actually encountered within clinical contexts.

Moreover, invoking patient autonomy as a kind of default position is akin to taking up the stance that patients and/or their families must be asked for their consent in every clinical ethics consultation situation. But as with the issue of consent, the question of who ought to participate turns on what is at stake for whom in actual clinical ethics consultation situations.

To begin to see how this notion of "what is at stake for whom" is a primary directive, again consider the fourth scenario, in which the focal theme is individuals' moral experience. In this kind of situation, careful inquiry into the actual details is often necessary as a means to appreciate the scope of moral considerations that confront the requestor (in that case, Stan Carmichel's burn physician). Learning these details may require that conversations occur with a number of individuals. In this scenario, this may likely include holding conversations with the chaplain, the ICU attending, members of the ICU nursing staff, if not also Stan's brothers. Since such conversations are for the sake of gaining the appropriate background, however, even if all of these individuals were to be gathered together in order to present to the HEC the history of the situation, the warrant for that gathering is not to be equated with what Stan's burn physician is asking of the HEC when she requests ethics consultation.

This physician understands and appreciates the perspectives of these other individuals involved in Stan's care; that is not her concern. But, we are told, she could not shake the feeling that backing off on Stan's interventions might not be the right thing to do. She is requesting ethics consultation to discuss questions *she* has regarding her *own* understanding and her *own* perspective. She is, in this sense, experiencing a kind of vulnerability as she struggles to make sense *for herself* what *matters to her*, such that she can take the next step (whatever it turns out to be) in her care of Stan. This physician's vulnerability cannot be ignored, for it is part of the core ethical question that has been put forward to the HEC. Actually answering the question of who ought to participate in the consultation with *her*, therefore, demands that such vulnerability be appreciated, evaluated, and taken into consideration.

In practice, this may mean any number of things. For instance, it may very well be that this physician would not only be made more vulnerable, but possibly even harmed, if she was asked to discuss openly her experience with these other individuals. This is not, of course, necessarily the case, and it might be that through a more communal discussion, she would receive needed support. Either may hold true, which highlights the fact that the question of participation is crucial and substantively significant for this physician.

The same, however, cannot be said in the circumstances involving Stan's brothers, the ICU physician, and the ICU nurses. For them, Stan's burn physician's understanding of her own moral commitments is primarily relevant in terms of the actions this physician has taken and will subsequently take. For example, imagine the perspective of Stan's brothers. Their aim is to prevent their brother from continuing to suffer under the burden of his injuries. In this aim, their goal is to have Stan's life-support removed, for him to be provided the appropriate palliative interventions, and to be allowed to die. If this goal requires Stan's burn physician to write an order saying this is what is to be done, then that is what they want. Their affiliation with Stan's burn physician is vested in their commitment toward Stan being treated in the manner they believe to be best for Stan. That commitment is what matters to them. As such, the burn physician's moral experience is not *directly* an issue for them except possibly in a certain kind of empathetic way. For them, the issue is having Stan cared for in the manner they believe appropriate. And in that concern, it is not relevant to them what this physician thinks or feels or perceives. For them, Stan's experience outweighs consideration of the physician's experience. This question of their participation in the ethics consultation, therefore, is relevant to them only if it helps achieve their aim, which differs from the concern of this physician (even if related via the potential action of withdrawing interventions from Stan).

A similar imaginative engagement may be directed toward the other individuals; for each, their aims and concerns, while tangentially related to those of Stan's burn physician, supercede how this physician understands her experience (except insofar as her understanding may have an effect on the achievement of their aims). As a result, if the aim of the consultation is to address the physician's concerns—which is what she has asked for—then the question regarding who ought to participate in this ethics consultation turns primarily on what will be most helpful for her in addressing the question, "Is the limiting or withdrawing of interventions the right thing to do here?" More generally, then, in ethics consultations primarily focused on concerns about moral experience, it may well be best to limit participation to just that one individual whose experience is raised for consideration, at least at first, in order to discover both the moral dimensions encountered by that individual and whether others should be involved. And this means the HEC must be prepared for having the option of no one else participating in the clinical ethics consultation.

Likewise, there may be reasons to include more participants and there may be reasons to include less when considering ethics consultations that direct attention on the relational dynamics involved in the patient-care situation. That determination will depend on the actual details of the clinical circumstances, what it is that prompts ethics consultation in the first place, and what turns out to be ethically at issue. For instance, consider the first two scenarios.

In the situation involving Janice Pear, her husband James has requested ethics consultation because he believes the nursing staff is trying to hasten his wife's death. There is any number of possible explanations regarding why he believes this. It may be that Mr. Pear is simply distraught over his wife's dying and he is directing his anguish toward the nurses. Or maybe he has misunderstood what Dr. McMillan stated during their meeting and so now misunderstands the nurses' recent actions. Or maybe, his belief accurately reflects that the night-shift nurse has disregarded the plan of care. Any of these may account for Mr. Pear's accusation against the nurses and thus his desire for ethics consultation. In order to address his concerns, however, the HEC will need to talk with Mr. Pear to discover which of these, or others, it is. In doing so, they will need to be cognizant that Mr. Pear *is* in the midst of watching his wife die, and hence may be especially vulnerable. They do not, therefore, want to construct a context for meeting and talking with him in which he may become further overwhelmed by the power and authority of the hospital, physicians, and so forth, which are so intertwined with the complexity of his recent experiences. At the same time, it is likely important that members of the care team, including Dr. McMillan, Dr. Worthington, Megan, and other representatives from the nursing staff, be available to join in the discussion in order to answer questions, to provide explanations, and possibly more important, to listen to what Mr. Pear has to say. Independent of what may be at stake for these care providers, their presence is one of the ways in which the HEC can demonstrate the seriousness with which it takes Mr. Pear's situation, and thus, is part of the effort to responsibly address what appears to be at stake for Mr. Pear such that he has requested ethics consultation.

At the same time, unbeknownst to the HEC at the time of request but possibly discovered in the process of addressing the explicit reason for ethics consultation, there may be important considerations associated with Dr. McMillan's response to not having been informed prior to the request that also need to be addressed (for instance, the scope and limit of nurses' responsibility). But such considerations do not concern Mrs. Pear's care per se. Indeed, it could be *any* patient and *any* family, and the particular medical situation could be any number of different kinds—and such considerations might still arise. All of the details associated with and specific to just this patient and family are, in other words, secondary to what is at stake in such considerations.

To address these (with all their complexities and implications concerning the life of the institution) requires a kind of focus different from what is raised when Mr. Pear, Dr. McMillan, Dr. Worthington, Megan, and others are invited to participate together in an examination of Mr. Pear's concerns. In fact, there is little warrant to have Mrs. Pear's family, Dr. Worthington, Megan, and staff nurses from the ICU involved. However, representatives from other aspects of the institution, such as nursing administration, would be required. What would be needed, in short, would be to create a forum in which Dr. McMillan and others could engage one another directly and specifically, without unnecessary constraint from the particulars of *this* clinical circumstance even though this clinical circumstance is what elicits these considerations at this time. The point here is to distinguish the issues that need to be clarified and discussed from the specific clinical events that bring them into focus. It is for this reason, then, that it may be better to limit participation when addressing considerations that supercede the particulars of the specific circumstance.

As for the scenario involving Mr. Freeman's family, the main issue revolves around tensions and complications in the relationship between and among Mr. Freeman's children, which raises a potential difficulty for the care providers as they try to determine where to send Mr. Freeman upon discharge. In this context, there is a clear need to have the children all together in order to ensure that whatever the internal politics of their family, the experience of those dynamics are, for the moment, put on hold in order for the HEC to help the care team figure out what is best for Mr. Freeman. As a result, there appears to be little warrant to have any other care providers participate except for Mr. Freeman's physician, especially since this physician had explicitly discussed Mr. Freeman's preferences with him several years prior. The role of this physician in the ethics consultation, however, is to help the family avoid getting caught up in its own dynamics and to help them instead place Mr. Freeman's care in the center of their concerns. What is at stake regards what is best for Mr. Freeman in view of his preferences, preferences that his children have also known for some time because Mr. Freeman had them participate in the drafting of his advance directive.

Each of the three scenarios discussed so far suggest the need for a different configuration of participants in the ethics consultation. All of this serves to confirm that it is the actual details of the clinical situation that are relevant for understanding and appreciating how the question of who ought to participate is to be answered.

The situation presented in the third scenario above is slightly different than the others, however, when considering the question of who ought to participate in an ethics consultation. The reason is that, unlike the other scenarios, in this one, identifying "what is at stake for whom" is not intimately dependent upon the kinds of details indicated in the previous scenarios. Rather, the details that matter are concerned more with the situation being of a particular kind than with individualistic matters. Recall, then, the situation presented in this scenario.

Dr. Roberts has questions about the status of a potential court order to provide transfusion to Rachel Williams, a minor who, along with her mother, has explicitly stated that she does not want blood products in light of her religious convictions (she is a Jehovah's Witness). Dr. Roberts has yet to decide whether she ought to transfuse Rachel; she recognizes, however, that *if* she decides to transfuse, a court order will be necessary. Accordingly, she is interested in making sure she understands the scope and limits associated with having a court order *should she request one*. In that concern, the particular details of this situation—that Rachel is the patient, that Rachel and her mother have expressed the preference not to be transfused, that some of the nurses and physicians involved in Rachel's care have voiced support for Rachel's preferences, that Dr. Roberts has yet to decide whether she'd transfuse Rachel—are not at stake; the reason is that the scope and limits of a court order granting legal permission to transfuse is per se independent of *these* details (details, it may be noted, that are of the kind that were relevant when considering the other scenarios).

To be sure, the issue of the court order serves as the focal point for a substantive question about what is best in this situation (even if that question is not immediately the one at hand). Moreover, pursuing the question of what is best in this situation includes the multiple senses of considering what is best for Rachel, for her mother, and for the medical and nursing staff as they provide care for Rachel and support for her parents. There is, then, a sense in which by seeking clarification about court orders, Dr. Roberts is not merely concerned with the legal reading per se; she is also concerned with how to ensure a supportive environment for Rachel in view of the potential legal implications associated with a potential court order. And this is *not* independent of Rachel, her parents, and so on, and so does appear to be intimately connected to the details of the situation.

And yet, even if Dr. Roberts is concerned with how to ensure a supportive environment for Rachel, it is not the substantive issue of whether transfusion is best for Rachel that is primarily at stake here; the primary issue is the substantive influence entailed by having a court order (whether or not it is actually invoked). Hence, for all these other individuals too—Rachel, her parents, the other care providers— the fact that there is a clear need to understand the scope and limits associated with having a court order is relevant, but not because of anything specific to them; they could be anyone. What is at stake here in having a court order, in other words, is not dependent upon the details of this situation. It is rather the way court orders function within clinical contexts and serve, so to speak, as part of the framework within which clinical care occurs. That it is *this* situation, with just *these* individuals participating is not, at the moment, the primary issue. Indeed, it could be any situation in which a court order potentially to allow intervention against the patient's or family's wishes may be sought, with any set of individuals serving in the various roles—patient, family, nurses, physicians—since the scope and limits of this kind of court order are the same regardless.

The fact that all of this is related to *this* situation may become relevant. But at this point, with Dr. Roberts's request for ethics consultation, the issue is one of the limits and scope of court orders in general. And this information is pertinent to all within the situation regardless of their particular biases regarding Jehovah's Witnesses and blood transfusions and Rachel's specific care. And, it is for that reason that all of the participants in this situation ought to participate in the ethics consultation. The more general point is that, due

to the fact that guidelines, policies, regulations, and so on, are neither more nor less specific to *any* of the particular participants involved in a specific situation, and thus relevant to *all* primary participants in that situation, when ethics consultation is requested for
these kinds of circumstances, the beginning stance should be that all
of the primary participants ought to be included in the ethics consultation process.

Who ought to participate in clinical ethics consultation is a question whose answer is neither easily nor singularly settled. Rather,
somewhat akin to the point made in the previous section—that it is
due to the actual circumstances of the specific clinical situation in
which ethics consultation occurs that informed consent may or may
not be fitting—what has been discussed in this section is meant to
demonstrate that the question of who ought to participate in clinical
ethics consultation primarily turns on dual considerations regarding
what is actually going on in the situation and what is at stake for the
potential participants, both for the situation generally and in the
ethics consultation more specifically. Accordingly, any individual's
participation is not to be rooted in the particular role occupied—
"patient," "family member," "physician," "nurse," and so on. As with
the issue of consent and ethics consultation, then, determining who
ought to participate must not betray those clinical elements that define that particular situation and give rise to those concerns for
which ethics consultation has been sought.

CONCLUSION

Much of the above discussion regarding consent for and participation in clinical ethics consultation is ultimately grounded in the
practical implications of the hallmark features of clinical contexts
mentioned in the introduction of this chapter, namely uncertainty,
ongoing change, forced trust, and the press of time. The reason, of
course, is that the practices of clinical ethics consultation, like the
practices of medicine and nursing, are bound by such features. Failure to appreciate these features does not negate their relevance or influence. The recognition that clinical ethics consultation is *clinical*
turns out to be crucial because HECs, like the individuals with whom
they interact, are faced with having to make real decisions, with actual consequences, in light of which many subsequent decisions and

actions (which are as yet unknown and still to come) gain meaning and merit.

As such, maintaining a stance that asserts that, for instance, consent is always necessary from patients or their families before clinical ethics consultation may proceed, or that everyone directly involved in a patient's clinical care ought to participate in the ethics consultation process, undercuts the very fabric that shapes the ethical dimensions of clinical care in the first place. The reason: such assertions and conclusions find their ground not in the dynamics of actual clinical life, but in the abstracted and constructed stances of academic or legalistic argument and position. However, for those who practice clinical ethics consultation, however, the demand of the actual details encountered within the real clinical circumstance for which ethics consultation has been requested are not mere constructs; they call for response, and for this reason, must be granted significant attention.

As a final note, it must be acknowledged that actually paying attention to the myriad of details present within any specific clinical circumstance is often no easy task. Accordingly, it may be difficult to determine just who ought to participate in a specific consultative episode and whether their consent should be pursued. However, disregarding such issues because they may be difficult to settle does not mitigate the need to engage in these kinds of determinations when serving as a clinical ethics consultant or member of an HEC (in the same way that ignoring the fact that clinical contexts are infused with uncertainty, undergo continual change, and so on, does not negate these facets). The moral grip of these questions is just one more reason why clinical ethics consultation must be approached and practiced with a healthy dose of humility and respect for the awesome responsibility of participating with others regarding matters of sickness and health, injury and recovery, life and death.

FOR FURTHER REFLECTION

1. In the section "Is Consent Required for Clinical Ethics Consultation?" it is suggested that while it may be reasonable for individuals to refuse to participate in an ethics consultation, their refusal cannot extend beyond their own participation; the process of ethics consultation may still move forward. Discuss how an ethics consultation might actually proceed if the individual

refusing is (a) the patient, (b) the patient's spouse, (c) the attending physician, or (d) the bedside nurse. Consider each of these first in the context of the four scenarios provided, and then in relation to the most recent ethics consultation in which you have been involved.

2. In response to the question of who ought to be included in an ethics consultation, the suggestion is that we begin with the perspective that all of the primary participants in the specific situation be included, and then, in light of both what is actually going on in that situation and what is morally relevant for those different primary participants, accommodations might need to be made. With this in mind, first, utilizing the four scenarios provided in this chapter, discuss what would have to have been different in each situation such that who might be included and who might be excluded in the ensuing ethics consultation could change. Second, do a similar exercise utilizing examples from your own ethics consultation experience. Finally, discuss actual ways in which you might prospectively evaluate whether patients, their family members, and medical and nursing staff ought to be included in ethics consultations.

NOTES

1. The question of participation in ethics consultation received some attention during the mid-1980s to early 1990s—mostly as part of broader discussions regarding the roles and functions of HECs (Randal 1983; Fost and Cranford 1985; Lo 1987; Cohen and d'Oronzio 1989; Stidham, Christensen, and Burke 1990; Agich and Youngner 1991)—before disappearing from the literature as discussion of clinical ethics consultation methodology and evaluation became more prominent.

2. There are likely numerous reasons why both the original question—whether patients can refuse ethics consultation—and the related concern—whether attending physicians need to give permission—have been addressed (or not) in the literature. What is more significant, however, is that both of these considerations share a similar presumption that, in light of even limited examination of the actual dynamics associated with clinical contexts, may be seen as problematic.

3. This represents a kind of irony, especially in relation to arguments for patients' having the option to consent to or refuse ethics consultation. The reason is that these arguments have all been rooted in the primacy of respecting patient autonomy, which itself is grounded in more fundamental considerations associated with the nature of being a person and belonging to a community of persons—not the roles individuals play (Faden and Beauchamp 1986, 235–73). More impor-

tantly, having a deep-seated commitment to the principle of respect for persons does not necessitate giving special dispensation to the individual whose autonomy bears respecting. In fact, the primary purveyors of this principle, Beauchamp and Childress, explicitly acknowledge that it is an error to equate demonstrating respect for one's autonomy with granting one's autonomy primacy over other considerations (and their implicit values) that might similarly be relevant in a given context (for example, community); "respect for autonomy," they state, "has only *prima facie* standing and can sometimes be overridden by competing moral considerations" (Beauchamp and Childress 2001). The point is that merely because individuals are due a certain respect of autonomy does not translate into their being given the right to determine what does, or does not, count as ethically relevant for others in a clinical situation.

WORKS CITED

Agich, G. J., and S. J. Youngner. 1991. For experts only? Access to hospital ethics committees. *Hastings Center Report* 21 (5): 17–25.

Arnold, R. M. 1994. Should competent patients or their families be notified before HECs review the patients' cases? Yes. *HEC Forum* 6 (4): 257–59.

Aulisio, M. P., R. M. Arnold, and S. J. Youngner, eds. 1999. Special issue: Commentary on the ASBH core competencies for health care ethics consultation. *The Journal of Clinical Ethics* 10 (1): 3–49.

Beauchamp, T. L., and J. F. Childress. 2001. *Principles of biomedical ethics*. 5th ed. New York: Oxford University Press.

Bemis, G. 1994. Should competent patients or their families be notified before HECs review the patients' cases? No. *HEC Forum* 6 (4): 262–65.

Bliton, M. J., and S. G. Finder. 1999. Strange, but not stranger: The peculiar visage of philosophy in clinical ethics consultation. *Human Studies* 22 (1): 69–97.

———. 2002. Traversing boundaries: Clinical ethics and moral experience in the withdrawal of life supports. *Theoretical Medicine* 23 (3): 233–58.

Cassell, E. J. 1991. *The nature of suffering and the goals of medicine*. New York: Oxford University Press.

Cohen, C. J., and J. C. d'Oronzio. 1989. The question of access. *HEC Forum* 1 (2): 89–103.

Faden, R. R., and T. L. Beauchamp. 1986. *A history and theory of informed consent*. New York: Oxford University Press.

Finder, S. G. 1995. Should competent patients or their families be able to refuse to allow an HEC case review? No. *HEC Forum* 7 (1): 51–53.

Fletcher, J. C. 1992. Ethics committees and due process. *Law, Medicine & Health Care* 20 (4): 291–93.

Fost, N., and R. E. Cranford. 1985. Hospital ethics committees: Administrative aspects. *New England Journal of Medicine* 253 (18): 2687–92.

LaPuma, J., C. B. Stocking, C. M. Darling, and M. Siegler. 1992. Community hospital ethics consultation: Evaluation and comparison with a university hospital service. *The American Journal of Medicine* 92:346–51.

Lo, B. 1987. Behind closed doors: Promise and pitfalls of ethics committees. *New England Journal of Medicine* 317 (1): 46–50.

Pellegrino, E. D. 1983. The healing relationship: The architechtonics of clinical medicine. In *The clinical encounter: The moral fabric of the physician patient relationship,* ed. E. E. Shelp. Dordecht and Boston: Reidel.

Perkins, H. S., and B. S. Saathoff. 1988. Impact of medical ethics consultation on physicians: An exploratory study. *The American Journal of Medicine* 85:761–65.

Purtilo, R. B. 1984. Ethics consultation in the hospital. *New England Journal of Medicine* 311(15): 983–86.

Randal, J. 1983. Are ethics committees alive and well? *Hastings Center Report* 13 (6): 10–12.

Roberts, L. W., T. McCarty, and G. B. Thaler. 1995. Should competent patients or their families be able to refuse to allow an HEC case review? Yes. *HEC Forum* 7 (1): 549–50.

Rubin, S., and L. Zoloth-Dorfman. 1994. First-person plural: Community and method in ethics consultation. *The Journal of Clinical Ethics* 5 (1): 49–54.

Simpson, K. H. 1992. The development of a clinical ethics consultation service in a community hospital. *The Journal of Clinical Ethics* 3 (2): 124–30.

Stidham, G. L, K. T. Christensen, and G. F. Burke. 1990. The role of patients/family members in the hospital ethics committee's review and deliberations. *HEC Forum* 2 (1): 3–17.

Veatch, R. M. 1989. Advice and consent. *Hastings Center Report* 19 (1): 20–22.

———. 2001. Ethics consultation: Permission from patients and other problems of methods. *American Journal of Bioethics* 1 (4): 43–45.

Wolf, S. M. 1991. Ethics committees and due process: Nesting rights in a community of caring. *Maryland Law Review* 50:798–858.

Zaner, R. M. 1988. *Ethics and the clinical encounter.* Englewood Cliffs, NJ: Prentice-Hall.

———. 1993. Voices and time: The venture of clinical ethics. *The Journal of Medicine and Philosophy* 18 (1): 9–31.

6

Cultural Diversity in the Clinical Setting

Alissa Hurwitz Swota

KEY POINTS

1. The importance of listening cannot be overemphasized.
2. Recognizing that there are differences in cultural practices and beliefs does not entail accepting all such practices and beliefs. It does necessitate trying to accommodate them in the absence of contraindications.
3. The ever-increasing amount of cultural diversity in the health-care context calls out for those working in such a setting to become culturally sensitive in order to provide optimal patient care.

The patient's beliefs, as well as body, must be treated.

—G. Galanti (2004), *Caring for Patients from Different Cultures*

Clashing cultural norms can contribute to the complex ethical terrain facing healthcare professionals and patients. Conflicts arising out of differences in cultural backgrounds are not surprising. Data from the U.S. Census Bureau show a "steady growth of ethnically diverse populations; from 12.3 percent in 1970, to 16.6 percent in 1980, to 19.7 percent in 2000," by the middle of this century, "ethnically diverse"[1] populations are anticipated to represent almost 50 percent of the population in the United States (Valle 2001). More specifically, practitioners can expect a patient population of which more than 40 percent are from "minority cultures" (American Medical Student Association 2005). These statistics serve to underscore the necessity for a greater level of cultural sensitivity in this "melting pot" society.

In this chapter, I will provide some insight into how and offer some specific examples of situations when the plurality of cultures in the clinical setting can lead to conflict.[2] I maintain that in order to decrease the likelihood and severity of conflicts fueled by cultural differences and achieve greater cooperation in the clinical context, health care professionals need to increase their levels of cultural sensitivity. In hopes of helping healthcare providers working amid the complex ethical terrain created by cultural pluralism, I will present some of the methodologies developed to aid in facilitating good communication, with the goal of building consensus around mutually agreeable treatment options.

CULTURE AND CULTURAL SENSITIVITY

For the sake of the following discussion, "culture" can be understood as encompassing "beliefs and behaviors that are learned and shared by members of a group" (Galanti 2004). It is a lens through which individuals view the world, affecting everything from what a person thinks illness is and how it is caused, to where decisional authority and control reside, "a 'context' within which one constructs ethical meaning"(Valle 2001). For instance, does an individual accept the notion of germ theory or does she believe that her disease was caused by evil spirits?[3] Is the patient the one who decides on a course of treatment, or is such a decision made by someone else in the family? Does the patient focus on the present or past, in contrast to the usually future-oriented perspective of Western[4] medicine? The answers to these questions will vary widely depending upon the "lens" through which one takes in the situation. In addition, the differences between healthcare providers and families do not end with culture, but are often compounded by differences in socioeconomic status, level of education, and individuality itself. As a result,

> what is known or valued by health care workers may be illusive or irrelevant to families. . . . Large health care teams with shifting and in-

consistent members—each trained in separate professions with separate working cultures—often fracture communication and make for an environment that is not conducive to balanced discussion and negotiation. (Bowman in press)

All of this lends support to the idea that those working within such large teams in a diverse healthcare setting need to aim toward becoming "culturally sensitive." Cultural sensitivity can be understood as being aware of one's own culture and the biases encompassed therein, being willing to understand and be open to the beliefs and practices of different cultures, and being willing to place an emphasis on communicating in a manner amenable to everyone involved. At the same time, being culturally sensitive does not mean accepting the relativistic view that whatever a person thinks is right or true for him or her is in fact right or true.[5] One can hold to a pluralistic view that acknowledges the importance of cultural beliefs, trying to work with them whenever possible, without having to accept the relativistic view that any and every cultural practice of all groups must be accepted.[6]

In the remainder of this section, I will take up some of the different aspects of cultural sensitivity that need to be addressed by healthcare practitioners—communication, whole-patient focus, and cultural-practice knowledge, in turn. Before discussing these and other issues, it is necessary to note that generalizations will be employed in achieving such ends—generalizations as opposed to stereotypes, as the former use information to identify common patterns within a group, leaving open the possibility that further data could show that the pattern is not applicable to a specific individual in a group, while the latter are used with no attempt made to see whether the pattern is in fact applicable to the individual (Galanti 2004). It cannot be stressed enough that each patient must be viewed as an individual who comes from a certain culture and who may or may not practice the traditions or hold the same beliefs and values as others in that culture. Cultures are not monolithic. Differences in factors such as age, socioeconomic status, and level of education and acculturation lend credence to the notion that variation among people from the same culture can often be as pronounced as variations between people from different cultures (see Muller and Desmond 1992). Practitioners need to view each patient as an individual. Part of that individual's identity is the cultural piece. However, how much or how little each individual subscribes to the dictates of her culture will vary from person to person. In short, the primary objective for the practitioner is to take care of the patient before him. Becoming culturally sensitive is instrumental in helping a provider provide the best patient care possible.

Overall, the generalizations in this chapter "are meant to be suggested guideposts, not precise, detailed maps. Ideally, they will help health care providers anticipate possibilities that should be considered, and make sense of behavior that has already occurred" (Galanti 2004). The use of generalizations is by no means meant to oversimplify the complexities surrounding cultural issues, but rather, it is meant to help *individuals* in the clinical setting deal with the issues openly and with sensitivity, and serve as a reminder that healthcare providers must

> continue the struggle to communicate complex and often frightening information across barriers of language and culture. [Health care providers] who dismiss the need for communication skills and a culturally sensitive approach to making medical decisions do so at the risk of providing substandard care.[7] (Powell 2006)

Achieving a greater level of cultural sensitivity can start with something as small as recognizing the importance of clear communication. In short, healthcare providers need to be able to understand the problem, both from a biomedical perspective and from the patient's perspective, if in fact the two diverge. In order to glean such an understanding, the healthcare provider needs at least to be able to solicit information from the patient, let the patient know that she may ask questions as well, and provide the patient with information. All of this presupposes the ability to communicate. Without such a foundation, the likelihood of a fruitful provider-patient relationship—to say nothing of a culturally sensitive approach to care—is minimal at best. The clinical setting is fast-paced, rife with complex terminology and confusing concepts that are new to many patients and families, and healthcare practitioners who have a limited amount of time for each patient and heavy workloads. Couple these conditions with the aforementioned fact that healthcare teams are often large and the communication therein fractured, and a diverse patient population some of whom have never interacted with the Western medical system, it is no wonder that miscommunications in the clinical context are not rare. What is surprising is that when miscommunications do occur, anyone is surprised.

Recognizing the need for clear communication can lead to concrete changes in the clinical setting—take, for example, an increase in the use of translators. Translators can help bridge the communication gap that might exist between patients and providers. In cases where one is uncertain, it is better to err on the side of caution and enlist the help of a translator. Sometimes the consequences of not using a translator when there is a question as to whether one is needed are tragic. For instance, a provider in Washington, DC, was sued for $11 million when, due to miscommunication, an abortion was performed on a non-English-speaking woman who only wanted contraceptive services (American Medical Student Association 2005). Though an extreme example, this case serves to highlight the severity of the consequences that may ensue when a translator is not used. In addition, not only are translators useful for their ability to make direct translations from one language to another, they can also help to clarify some of the cultural differences that might exist (Juckett 2005).

Individuals used to translate may include, but are not limited to, those who are specially trained to translate within the clinical context, individuals who do translating but have not been trained to work specifically within the clinical context, someone on staff who speaks the language at issue, or a family member or friend of the patient.[8] To be sure, in using a family member or friend as a translator, one runs many risks (see Juckett 2005). For example, the translator might not tell the patient about a terminal diagnosis. This could be attributed to a number of different reasons including a lack of comfort in being the bearer of such news or wanting to protect the patient from an unpleasant diagnosis. In addition, if the situation is one in which a younger member of the family is translating for an older member of the family,[9] there are a variety of different health issues that might be seen as "improper" subjects for discussion (for example, a son translating for his mother concerning gynecological health problems). When using medical personnel within the institution, there is a potential for patients and families to perceive a conflict of interest—namely, that the translator might manipulate the information he conveys in order to achieve the best outcome for the hospital. Given the potential hazards of using family members as translators, and the possibility of a conflict of interest (whether it be real or merely perceived) when using medical personnel, it looks as though the best practice, both in terms of cultural sensitivity and ethics, is to employ "outside" translators.[10] With phone translating services available at all times of the day (for a fee), the option of utilizing a formal translator has become a bit more real for institutions that previously had limited access.[11]

In addition, to deal with conflicts in clinical contexts, providers and consultants must recognize the influence cultural beliefs have on how one cares for and understands the body. As a result, successful treatment of patients means taking "their beliefs into account, whether they are about the causes of disease, how it should be treated, what behavior is appropriate, or how the body is to be viewed" (Galanti 2004). Cultural sensitivity entails recognizing cultural differences not as barriers to providing health care, but as integral in providing care for the *whole* patient.[12] As such, cultural sensitivity can be viewed not merely as something that it would be good to aspire to, but instead, as an integral component of quality health care. For example, rather than dismissing a request from a Native American patient to have a traditional healer come in to perform a healing ritual, a culturally sensitive provider might discuss the intricacies of the ritual to see if anything is contraindicated. In the absence of any contraindications, reasonable accommodations to allow for the performance of the ritual should be made (Berger 1998). This willingness to merge traditional Western medicine with practices and traditions of other cultures is a necessity in our pluralistic society.

Based on consequentialist reasons alone, it is clear that an increase in our level of cultural sensitivity is imperative. In terms of consequences, the results of a lack of attention to cultural diversity have been devastating. In one case, a "Vietnamese father who had treated his son with coin rubbing (*cao gio*) committed suicide in jail after mistakenly being accused of child abuse based on the marks on the boy" (Flores et al. 2002). Coin rubbing is a practice common to many Asian cultures. It is employed to "relieve fever, headache and chills . . . [and involves] rubbing the edge of a coin against the skin until a purpuric or petechial rash appears" (Rosenblat and Hong 1989). While marks on a child may flag the possibility of child abuse, a culturally sensitive approach would consider other possible explanations as well. Had the healthcare providers been more familiar with traditional folk treatments (or, at least, more willing to engage the family in discussions of cultural healing practices), this tragic situation might have been avoided.

UNDERSTANDING AUTONOMY

Crucial to respecting patients in Western medicine is making sure that efforts are made to recognize and promote patient autonomy. Though reverence toward autonomy is not as absolute as it was just a few years ago, the present assumption under which those in Western medicine operate continues to be that "autonomy is king." As Renee Fox notes, "[F]rom the outset, the conceptual framework of bioethics has accorded paramount status to the value-complex of individualism, underscoring the principles of individual rights, autonomy, self-determination, and their legal expression in the jurisprudential notion of privacy" (as cited in Macklin 2006). In theory, a strong emphasis on autonomy is compatible with a conception of shared decision making, but in practice, respect for autonomy has been taken to mean that individuals are entitled to, or even obligated to, make their own medical decisions. More specifically, the Western conception of the patient is one of an individual who has a future-oriented perspective and wants to be told truthful information about her diagnosis in order to make an informed decision about her medical treatment plan (Marshall et al. 1998). This individualistic conception of patients, with an emphasis on autonomy and an underlying assumption that people want to play an active role in medical decision making, is quite positive in many ways. Historically, such a role had been withheld from people, especially within the medical setting, for too long. Empowering patients and giving more weight to patient autonomy was heralded as the means by which patients would be guaranteed a role in the decision-making process and a chance to continue to incorporate their values in deciding how to live their lives.

However, when such a conception of the patient is adopted to the exclusion of all others, when the understanding of the very complex concept of autonomy is too narrow, one is left with an impoverished view that cannot function in a diverse clinical setting or account for the plurality of views therein. The case below serves to underscore the importance of taking on a robust conception of autonomy in the clinical setting:

Mr. Okimoto is an eighty-two-year-old Japanese man with metastatic esophageal cancer. Over the past few months, it has become quite hard for him to eat by mouth. He has lost a great deal of weight and appears emaciated. In order to get a sufficient number of calories, it is suggested that Mr. Okimoto receive a feeding tube. Placing the tube will provide better nutrition and thus give Mr. Okimoto more time (likely measured in months) and not decrease his quality of life too much. Mr. Okimoto's family has been at his side throughout his long struggle. This has meant that many of his children have had to fly across country and have been missing work and their own families in order to be with him during his time of need. Economic costs, though real, pale in comparison to the emotional toll this long illness has taken on his family. Mr. Okimoto believes he has become a burden to his family. This is something that Mr. Okimoto never wanted to see happen. Ultimately, Mr. Okimoto refuses to have the feeding tube placed. The attending physician becomes quite concerned and believes that Mr. Okimoto's family might be pressuring him to give up and refuse beneficial treatment. A consult is called by the physician who has relayed his concerns to the whole healthcare team and raised the level of anxiety for everyone involved in the case.

Though the physician's concern is well intentioned, it comes out of a view that understands autonomy in a very narrow sense. On such a view, the great weight Mr. Okimoto gives to the impact a treatment choice has on his family verges on a sort of coercion or undue influence, which could interfere with Mr. Okimoto's autonomy. Such a conception of autonomy fails to recognize that a decision that takes into account the well-being of others is no less likely to be autonomous than one that does not. The question of whether the patient has acted autonomously is not answered by looking at whether the decision was made in isolation, without any outside influences.[13] This atomistic conception lies in stark contrast to a view of the patient as part of a larger unit. Whether such a unit is a nuclear or extended family, a tribe, a clan, or something else entirely, it provides the context within which the individual views herself and from which she finds meaning and value. In short, the physician's perspective concentrates too much on Mr. Okimoto as divorced from his context and fails to recognize the significance that "other-directed" concerns can play in an autonomous decision-making process.[14]

In addition, during the ethics consult with the healthcare team, Mr. Okimoto, and the Okimoto family, it is explained that Mr. Okimoto is a Buddhist, and "Buddhist thought emphasizes compassion and justice. Patients who forgo life-sustaining treatment so that the family does not suffer, emotionally or financially, are performing a valued act of compassion" (Berger 1998).[15] Far from being coerced into refusing the feeding tube, Mr. Okimoto chooses such a treatment plan and does so without hesitation or undue influence, believing that he has chosen to act justly and with care and concern for his beloved family. And, though the physician was only trying to make sure that Mr. Okimoto's autonomy was respected, had he taken a more robust view of autonomy and considered Mr. Okimoto as part of a larger whole, tensions may not have gotten so high and the trust between the healthcare team and the family may not have been put to such a test. In the clinical context, autonomy is displayed in a variety of ways. As such, a broad construal of autonomy needs to be maintained in order for it to hold any real meaning and be able to function in a pluralistic clinical setting.

TRUTH-TELLING

The autonomy-focused Western conception of the patient lies in opposition to many cultures in which the patient is viewed as part of a greater whole, the family unit, rather than as a discrete individual. In these other cultures the truth about a diagnosis may likely not be given directly to the patient, nor would the patient want or expect such information. To be sure, a mere fifty years ago, the concealing of the truth that is currently standard in other cultures, was an integral part of Western medicine. Today, standard practice in Western medicine is to give patients information concerning diagnosis and treatment options so as to enable them to make informed decisions.[16] To do otherwise might seem wrong, contrary to professional and institutional standards at least, and perhaps dishonest and morally blameworthy. Providing information to patients is seen not only as a way to respect their autonomy, but not to do so, to withhold information from them, is seen as a harm, an affront to their dignity and capacity to act as rational agents. However, it is quite dangerous to assume that everyone subscribes to the same values and beliefs. The idea that everyone gives primacy to autonomy and considers it a harm to withhold the truth about a diagnosis from patients is a particularly Western notion.

In their study, Blackhall et al. (2001) note that most of the African American and European American respondents held the more traditional Western view that places primacy on autonomy and the provision of information to the individual patient in order to enable her to make a treatment decision based on her own values. Alternately, most of the Mexican American and Korean American respondents viewed patients not so much as individuals, but more so, as but one part of a "social network" (Blackhall et al. 2001).[17] This cleavage between cultures regarding the prioritization and weighting of different values is not surprising. Valle (2001), through a compilation of studies, does a nice job comparing what a hierarchy of bioethical principles would look like from a "mainstream" Western perspective, versus an "ethnically diverse" perspective (that is, a perspective different from the one of traditional Western medicine). The results of this comparison show the "mainstream" Western perspective placing autonomy at the top of the list followed by truth-telling, beneficence, nonmaleficence, and distributive justice in descending order (Valle 2001). Ranking on the "ethnically diverse" perspective looks quite a bit different, with beneficence at the top of the list followed by nonmaleficence, distributive justice, autonomy, and truth-telling in descending order (Valle 2001). Of note is the placement of truth-telling near the top of the list from a "mainstream" perspective, and at the bottom of the list on an "ethnically diverse" perspective.

Contrary to a traditional Western perspective, with both Mexican Americans and Korean Americans (among others), it is often held that more harm is done by telling the patient the truth. Telling a patient the truth about a grave condition in these latter cultures can be seen as taking hope away from the patient—a great harm since life without hope is of substandard quality at best, and at worst, not worth living at all. These differences serve to illustrate that in trying to respect the values held by others and abide by the basic imperative "do no harm," itself a dictum native to Western medicine, one might not have an easy time of it. Harm can be interpreted in vastly different ways, which are determined, in large part, by the worldview with which one comes to the table. As one study notes, "Statistical analysis of the data, controlling for variables such as income, education, and access to care, revealed that ethnicity was the most important factor contributing to attitudes toward truth-telling" (Blackhall et al. 2001). By implication, the magnitude of the harm (or lack thereof) done when the truth is withheld is also a function of one's culture.

Specific concerns that are noted when there is a question as to whether to tell an individual the truth about her medical treatment include the worry that not to tell someone the truth would be to deprive her of the ability to plan (at least with any accuracy) her remaining time.[18] Specifically, one would not be able to consider final arrangements including people to see, things to say, and items to give to others in person. In addition, one might miss the opportunity to make sure certain things are put in writing and determine where to be when death occurs (for example, at home, in a foreign country, in another state with family, and so forth). To be sure, the edifice upon which these concerns are built is constructed with a focus found in a Western perspective, namely, the idea that control should be vested in the individual. This focus runs contrary to many cultures where control is distributed among family or clan and shared decision making is the norm, with primary concern placed on how the decision will affect others. Such a concern, though present in Western culture, is commonly not given primacy over the idea that the individual should be the one making the decision.

Doing double duty, the next case serves to highlight how different cultures can place truth-telling and patient autonomy at vastly different levels of import and the danger of using family members as translators.[19]

> Mrs. Chen is an eighty-four-year-old Chinese woman who speaks very little English. She has metastatic cancer, and her prognosis is quite grim. She lives with her son, and he has always served as her translator. By all accounts from the healthcare team, Mrs. Chen knows that she has cancer and that her time is limited. Her physician explained that he told her himself, using Mrs. Chen's son to translate. One day a nurse is in the room and mentions something about the cancer diagnosis. Mrs. Chen is clearly shocked and sinks into a deep depression. When he arrives later that day, Mrs. Chen's son is outraged that the nurse would tell his mother about the cancer diagnosis. The nurse feels awful about upsetting Mrs. Chen. At the same time, she and other members of the healthcare team are confused, since they were under the impression that Mrs. Chen was aware of her diagnosis and prognosis. However, Mrs. Chen's son had not been translating exactly what the doctor said. In fact, not only had he not told his mother of her poor prognosis, he never told her that she had cancer. He saw his role as protector of his mother and thought that if he told her the truth about her condition, he would devastate her and remove all hope and possibility of enjoyment during her last days and months.[20]

For Mrs. Chen's son to define his role as protector and to hold that protection entails withholding such a grim prognosis from his mother is not surprising given the culture with which he identifies and in light of the ranking of values noted earlier. As one study noted, "Duty was defined by both Latino and Chinese relatives as protecting the patient

. . . by making the remaining time comfortable and free of distress. Central to the concept of protection was a need to keep information about disease and prognosis from the patient" (Marshall et al. 1998). Reticence in telling a patient the truth about a grim diagnosis is also common to the Japanese and Navajo culture. In fact, in the latter two cultures, merely broaching the topic of terminal prognosis is seen, in a sense, to hasten death (Berger 1998). The strength of this belief is made clear in a study which found that only 13 percent of physicians in Japan said that they would tell their patient about a cancer diagnosis (Berger 1998).

Another reason given for not informing a patient about a poor prognosis is that there is no reason to tell a patient something that she probably already knows. To be sure, such knowledge, if it exists at all, is most likely at a very general level, and what the specific medical problem is remains unknown to the patient. The claim, however, is simply that it is enough that the patient knows that she has *some* problem, and if she wants further information she will ask for it when she is ready. It is not up to her healthcare providers to divulge such information unsolicited. As Blackhall et al. found, common across European American, African American, Korean American, and Mexican American respondents is the idea that withholding information from a patient is not likely to guarantee that the patient will not know the truth (Blackhall et al. 2001). Common to members of all of these groups was the assumption that the patient already knows that something is wrong; it is what drove her to go to the doctor in the first place (Blackhall et al. 2001). For African Americans and European Americans, this knowledge buttresses an obligation on the part of healthcare providers to tell the patient exactly what is wrong and make sure that the patient is an informed participant in the medical treatment plan. When couched within a Korean American or Mexican American population, this same idea, that the patient already knows that something is wrong, translates into a reason *not* to tell the patient the truth because to do so would be to force her to face what she already knows and what she would ask about if she in fact did desire more information. Of note here is the fact that the same insight, that patients usually know that something is wrong with them in the first place, warrants two vastly different calls to action based on the cultural lens through which one is looking at the situation.

Culturally sensitive healthcare providers recognize that "effective, culturally sensitive communication is a necessary part of providing high quality care" (Powell 2006). As such, they work toward determining what "good disclosure" looks like to the patient, asking questions like, how much information is sufficient to disclose in order to satisfy the patient's needs? How much would be too much for the patient to handle? How often should the subject be revisited to ensure that the patient's preferences have not changed? In general, when it comes to relating a grim diagnosis to a patient, one needs to "be restrained in relating bad news or explaining in detail complications that may result from a particular course of treatment. In many cultures, placing oneself in the doctor's hands represents an act of trust and a desire to transfer the responsibility for treatment to the physician" (American Medical Student Association 2005). While one is conveying such information, there is a need to be vigilant and make sure that the patient is not being overloaded with information she is not able to handle. The healthcare provider, in attempting to get the information across to the patient, must take care to do so at a pace and level that is appropriate to and dictated by the patient, focusing on both substance and process.[21] As far as how much information is appropriate to give to a patient, "the fullest understanding of the disease the patient can tolerate" is a good level at which to aim (Marshall et al. 1998).

In addition, even though a patient may come from a culture that emphasizes beneficence over autonomy and places decision-making authority in the hands of the family as opposed to the patient, one cannot and *must* not assume that the patient subscribes to these same ideals.[22] [23] If the patient wants information regarding her condition, even if her family says no, the patient's preferences and right to information are to be respected over the protests and preferences of her family.[24] Alternatively, the patient might choose to exercise her autonomy with a different end in mind, namely, not to be informed of the details of her medical condition and treatment. In cases where a patient chooses not to be fully informed about her condition, providers must still obtain an informed consent (or an informed refusal) for treatment, and this is quite possible within the framework of U.S. law.[25] Since one of the main functions of informed consent is to help ensure patient autonomy is respected, there is a worry that not to give patients information regarding their condition is tantamount to not respecting their autonomy. Such a worry is not well founded, as respect for patient autonomy is manifested in a variety of ways. For instance, if a healthcare provider approaches a patient and tells her that he has information regarding her condition, it is perfectly acceptable to agree to a request from the patient not to give her any information regarding her condition, and instead, have her spouse handle everything. This attempt at providing the patient with information should be noted in the chart, along with a mention of how the healthcare provider made sure that the patient was aware that she was refusing such information, that it would be given instead to the person she designated, and that it was made clear to the patient that information is available to her at any time in the future if she changes her mind. Further, verification that the patient has not changed her mind should be sought through future attempts at offering her information. Charting that such attempts have been made every couple of days,[26] and noting whether the patient has had a change of heart, will help the healthcare team to keep track of patient preferences. This informed decision to not receive information is as autonomous as a decision to be given any and all information. Consent in such a case should be obtained from the individual named by the patient to receive such information. In other words, "A patient's right to information is respected no less when the patient chooses to be relatively uninformed as when full information is demanded" (Hern et al. 1998).[27] In either case, healthcare professionals need to be sure to make it clear that information is available to the patient whenever she would like, that every reasonable effort will be made to accommodate her preferences, and that everyone involved has the same goal—making sure that the patient receives excellent care.

ADVANCE CARE PLANNING AND CARE AT THE END OF LIFE

One useful example of an area of health care where extra caution must be taken, especially in light of cultural differences and the potential for conflict, is advance care planning and care at the end of life. With the passing of the Patient Self-Determination Act (PSDA) in 1990, it became mandatory for all hospitals and healthcare providers reimbursed by Medicare or Medicaid to inform patients, upon admission, about advance directives and their rights regarding these documents. The PSDA, among other things, buttressed the existing support for patient autonomy. As advance directives provide a vehicle through which an individual can retain a voice in her medical fate even after she no longer has decisional capacity, patient autonomy is thus extended. This desire to enable individuals to maintain control accords with the previous description of the values entrenched within Western medicine and the revered position it grants to autonomy. However, not all cultures share the same attitude about the documents. And, as one study noted, "ethnicity was the second most significant predictor of possession of an advance directive after education" (Berger 1998).[28] In another study, "only 25% of the African-American population, compared to 86% of the Euro American population, reported a desire to complete an advance directive" (Marshall et al. 1998). When Navajo patients, health providers, and traditional healers were surveyed, "86% of the individuals interviewed considered discussion of advance care planning for near-death medical decisions a dangerous violation of Navajo values" (Marshall et al. 1998). Thus, while a Western perspective holds advance directives in high regard for their role in respecting patient autonomy, other cultures believe that to even talk about the issues often covered in these directives (e.g., illness and dire prognoses), is tantamount to causing them to come to fruition. In general, "advance directives presuppose a very particular conception of the self, or what it means to be a person. . . . for example, that persons, even in the face of death, are and ought to be 'rational', that, even in the face of death, persons want to speak and hear the truth about their condition, and that persons largely want to make treatment decisions by and for themselves" (Parens 1998).[29] Thus, when engaging in advance care planning (and medical treatment decision making in general), "health care professionals should remember that many patients have immigrated from countries where as much as three-fourths of the population does not have access to basic health needs. . . . They have never before faced 'high-tech' health care," and often do not have a clear understanding of what to expect from various medical treatment options (Klessig 1992).

Being sensitive to the multiple attitudes concerning advance care planning can help to avoid some of the tension and confusion like that encountered in the following case:

Mrs. Pierce is a seventy-four-year-old Navajo woman. She has lived with her son and his family for the last five years. She is a diabetic and presents with dizziness and general malaise. On admission to the hospital clinic, Mrs. Pierce and her son are given some information concerning advance directives. While the physician was reading her chart, he noted her age and that her chronic condition had worsened quite a bit over the past couple of years. In light of this deterioration, the doctor thought it was a good time to talk about advance care planning, using the materials that Mrs. Piece had already received. Shortly after beginning to discuss advance directives in detail, Mrs. Pierce and her son became anxious and agitated. Security had to be called after they began yelling at the physician.

From the perspective of the physician, no wrong was done to cause such an emotional outburst. Far from doing harm, he thought that he was doing a good thing by taking time out to discuss treatment options that could be included in an advance directive (with her specific condition in mind) and making sure that Mrs. Pierce would receive care that she deemed appropriate in case she became incapacitated and was not able to speak for herself. The physician was amazed that Mrs. Pierce and her son would be so unappreciative and combative. Conversely, Mrs. Pierce and her son found the physician's talk about treatment options in case of grim prognoses to be disrespectful and irrelevant. It was disrespectful because "in Navajo culture, an important concept is 'Hozho' that involves goodness, harmony, positive attitude, and universal beauty. Negative thoughts of illness raised in discussions of advance health planning conflict with this philosophy" (Berger 1998).[30] Moreover, since those in the Navajo culture are often "present-oriented," any talk of *advance* care planning and a potentially grim future is "culturally irrelevant" (Berger 1998).

How then can advance care planning and care at the end of life be approached so as to minimize the chance of conflict and misunderstanding? In non-Western cultures, decision making is often family-centered as opposed to resting with the individual patient. As such, if there is an indication that advance care planning is a topic that may be broached, bringing in the family (with the patient's permission) during the process may help to facilitate things.[31] This process must proceed slowly, with the patient and the patient's family setting the pace. Frequent pauses for questions and for allowing the patient and family to put the process on hold are a good idea. One might even frame the potential illnesses and treatments in terms of them happening to someone else, or talking about certain conditions in the abstract as opposed to befalling the patient (Jecker et al. 1995).

It might also be useful to talk about what is important to the patient, framing questions in terms of what is of value to the patient as opposed to mentioning specific diseases and illnesses and various poor conditions. This will give insight into the outcomes in terms of quality of life that the patient would and would not find acceptable and provide guidance in determining a treatment plan when and if the patient can no longer speak for herself. After determining the goals of treatment from the patient's perspective, it is useful to discuss whether such goals can be achieved. If not, investigation into alternative goals ought to be pursued. Overall, when engaging in advance care planning and decision making at the end of life, one needs to proceed with caution, making sure to treat each situation as unique, with the ultimate goal of providing good patient care. The following table offers a rough sketch of Western versus non-Western views on some general end-of-life issues, which provide some rules of thumb for health care professionals (see Table 6.1).

COMMUNICATION STRATEGIES

There will be conflicts in the clinical setting that are driven, in large part, by cultural differences. There is no way to know everything about every culture (including one's own).[32] Given this recipe for potential strife, the following are some things to keep in mind when negotiating the intricate terrain created by the plurality of cultures that abound in the clinical setting. Though no single method is guaranteed to avoid or resolve conflicts, one thing that must always be emphasized is a focus on open communication from all parties and creating an environment of trust that is hospitable to posing questions and investigating and negotiating differences. Often, simply acknowledging differences will lead to improved communication (Bowman in press).

When a hospital ethics committee (HEC) is called in to consult, the conflict is often already quite intense. In addition to gathering as much information as possible about the case before meeting with the involved parties, HEC members must be vigilant during the meeting, recognizing that just as the patients and their families come to the table with their own perspectives and values, so too do the healthcare providers and the consultants. Acknowledgment of these differences can have a profound effect on the situation. Making it

Table 6.1. General Views on End-of-Life Issues

	Contemporary Medical Perspectives	Non-Western Perspectives	Clinical Approach
Beliefs about causation of death and dying	Biologically determined. Dying occurs when medicine can no longer stave off, treat, or reverse illness. Death most often occurs in hospitals, and the declaration of death is ultimately in the hands of medical personnel.	Death may be seen in a broader and seemingly less tangible manner. May be viewed as being linked to religious, social, spiritual, and environmental determinants. Some cultural groups may perceive illness and death as separate entities. Declaration of death is also socially and culturally determined.	Anticipate nonmedical perspectives on death. Allow cultural rituals. Allow flexibility with time spent with the dying or deceased. Explore perceptions about the causes of the critical illness, its treatment, and death.
Communicating about dying to patients and others	Information explicitly communicated. Moral obligation to truth-telling as patient has right to know and must make autonomous decisions. Information best overtly communicated.	Moral duty to protect loved ones from negativity. Cues taken from the social context. Frank communication about death often unacceptable. Truth-telling highly problematic.	Ask patient how much medical information he/she wishes to have. Ask how information should be communicated.
Perception of negotiating death (levels of negotiating treatment)	Patients are largely responsible for defining the "kind of death" they wish.	Suffering and death are largely a matter of fate and may hold profound spiritual meaning.	Trial of therapy allows patient outcomes to be determined more by "fate."
Timing of death	The timing and circumstances of death can and ought to be controlled as much as possible to respect a patient's autonomous choices.	The timing and circumstances of death and dying are preordained and a matter of fate.	Allow as natural a process as possible. If on life support, withdraw gradually.

Note: For entire chart, see Kerry Bowman, *Understanding and Respecting Cultural Differences in End-of-Life Care*, in press.

clear that these different perspectives, values, and traditions are present, and that every attempt will be made to respect them, can, at the very least, have a cathartic effect and potentially play a pivotal role in resolving the conflict. Hopefully, patients will be comfortable enough to take a leading role in directing the conversation, with healthcare professionals making sure to go beyond simply hearing the patient and engage in active listening. For instance, the healthcare practitioner should give the patient his undivided attention, acknowledging with nonverbal cues, when appropriate, what the patient is saying. It is often useful for the practitioner, in his own words, to repeat back to the patient what she has told you. This provides an opportunity to clarify communication and correct any misunderstandings that might be present. The importance of listening cannot be overemphasized. Having the training and knowledge to pick up on clues and act on information the patient and the patient's family provides will increase the likelihood of a successful interaction. Hopefully, the following models will provide a start for such training and a strong foundation upon which to build in becoming culturally sensitive.

The following eight questions, developed by Arthur Kleinman et al., can help healthcare providers survey the landscape and determine how patients and their families view illness. Ideally these questions will assist providers in beginning a dialogue to recognize differences, in hopes of both avoiding conflicts, and resolving them if they have already developed:

1. What do you call the problem?
2. What do you think has caused the problem?
3. Why do you think it started when it did?
4. What do you think the sickness does?
5. How severe is the sickness? Will it have a short or long course?
6. What kind of treatment do you think the patient should receive? What are the most important results you hope she receives from this treatment?
7. What are the chief problems the sickness has caused?
8. What do you fear most about the sickness? (as cited in Galanti 2004)

Eliciting the answers to these questions can be seen at least as an act in good faith to try to understand all perspectives brought to the situation, and at most, can serve to resolve conflicts that at first blush seemed intractable. Additional insight can be gleaned by keeping the following considerations in mind:

- determination of the language used by patients and families to discuss their disease;
- elicitation of the patient's and family's understanding of the cause of and best treatment of the illness;
- consideration of the influence of gender and age;
- determination of who is considered to be the appropriate decision maker (including the option of joint, consensual decision making);
- consideration of religious beliefs;
- and recognition of broader political and historical context that might impact patient care, such as unequal access to services or discrimination. (Marshall et al. 1998)

All of these factors play into how one views illness, and thus, how one views treatment and the decision-making process involved in determining a treatment plan.

In the end, a culturally sensitive individual in the clinical setting will listen with the goal of understanding not only the "whats" and "hows" of other cultures, but also the "whys." In kind, an explanation of the pertinent components of a Western model, why we do things and what we expect from doing them, should be offered. The idea of gaining understanding as a process as opposed to an event will allow for expectations to be set at a reasonable level. That is, healthcare providers should not expect to come away with all of the knowledge and insight needed to make a thoughtful decision after one brief encounter. Necessary components for the intricate work involved in negotiating cross-cultural differences are an open mind; an environment of trust; strong, open lines of communication; and a lot of patience. Creativity and ingenuity are also valuable attributes when developing options around which consensus can be built. Moreover, careful attention must be paid to making sure that everyone has been heard and has been a part of the decision-making process. As a result, everyone will have partial "ownership" of the decision, making it easier to accept than if they have a treatment plan, the development of which they were not a part, thrust upon them. Of equal importance is the notion that no one can go into a conflict-ridden situation owning a particular result; to do so would lead to someone being the "loser" and someone else being the "winner."[33] That is far from the type of attitude that can lead to developing consensus around mutually acceptable treatment options. Oftentimes, negotiation involves entertaining different ways of interpreting the principles that guide your decision making, those points by which you set your own moral compass. In some instances, it will become clear that you can arrive at mutually agreeable treatment plans; at other times, no compromise reveals itself. Becoming a culturally sensitive healthcare provider means being aware of and open to different interpretations of data and different methods of treatment, and realizing that even when no compromise can be found, much can be learned in the process.

FOR FURTHER REFLECTION

1. Given the importance of becoming culturally sensitive, what can hospitals do to increase the level of cultural sensitivity of their healthcare providers?
2. Ought there to be cultural sensitivity requirements (for example, competency tests) for healthcare providers?
3. Though not focused on in this chapter, another important example of how differences in cultural practices are manifested is in terms of different practices of handling the recently deceased. How might a culturally sensitive provider deal with an Iranian family who insists that their loved one, who died from an unknown pathogen that poses a potential public-health threat, be buried within forty-eight hours?

NOTES

Thank you to Bonnie Steinbock and Mitch Haney for help on early versions of this piece.

1. That is, "ethnically diverse" as opposed to "mainstream Euro ethnic groups" (Valle 2001).
2. Here I am referring to the fact that there are a number of different cultures in our society, and by implication, in our healthcare system. I am assuming that within such a varied society and clinical setting, we want to maximize cooperation. As such,

we ought to strive to become culturally sensitive (as I will later define it) as one means by which we can achieve greater cooperation. For an extended discussion on maximizing cooperation in a pluralistic society in general, see John Rawls (1971), *A Theory of Justice*. For a thoughtful, in-depth discussion on pluralism, see John Kekes (1996), *The Morality of Pluralism*.

3. Oftentimes, Western medicine and traditional healers can work together to treat individuals who "see a medical doctor for relief of symptoms while also going to a folk doctor or traditional healer to be rid of the cause of illness" (American Medical Student Association 2005). To be sure, the belief one has in the power of one's respective cultural practices can play a pivotal role in the attitude with which one faces illness and the potential success of treatment.

4. I am aware that the term "Western" is problematic in itself. In this chapter, I use it as shorthand for a number of different groups. As such, it may at times confound several cultural groups, including but not limited to, North Americans, European Americans, and Afro-Americans.

5. There are several criticisms of ethical relativism. For a succinct discussion of some of the criticisms of ethical relativism, see Jecker et al. (1995), chapter 2 herein, as well as Steinbock et al., 2003.

6. For a more extended discussion of this point, see Jecker et al. (1995), chapter 2 herein, and Macklin 2006.

7. Bracketed sections are my emendation.

8. In March of 2006, it was announced that a computer system had been developed that helps healthcare professionals talk to their patients in different languages. The system is already being used in limited areas in the United States and Canada (CBC 2006). See Haffner (1992) for a firsthand account of some of the issues involved in translating in the medical setting.

9. Here I am referring specifically to intergenerational translation.

10. Ideally the "outside" translator will be able to be present, but formal translators accessed via telephone would still be preferable to family members and hospital personnel.

11. Only two states in the United States currently provide third-party reimbursement for interpreter services (Flores et al. 2002).

12. The importance of treating not just the physical, but also the psychological and social aspects of the patient has foundations rooted in the work of Paul Ramsey (*The Patient as a Person*, 1970) as well as George Engel's "biopsychosocial" model of health care (1977), and is well argued by Edmund Pelligrino in *The Anatomy of Clinical Judgments: Some Notes on Right Reason and Right Action* (1979).

13. In this case, the physician views *any* influence as infringing on patient autonomy.

14. See Hester (2001) for a detailed discussion of how engaging the patient as a participant in his or her medical treatment entails understanding the patient as a member of a larger community.

15. In this case, the patient's beliefs about what is compassionate and just are grounded in a well-known belief system—Buddhism. This tie to Buddhism is provided merely as additional background information. That is, it is not in virtue of the fact that Mr. Okimoto's preferences are grounded in a well-known belief system that provides necessary or sufficient conditions for respecting such beliefs. Indeed,

healthcare professionals ought to be open to accepting any number of reasoned conceptions of what is compassionate and just.

16. Truth-telling is a great example of a case where there seem to be at least two different dimensions to differing values and attitudes—a temporal as well as a cultural (geographical) dimension. This makes it more difficult to know whether the difference in values and attitudes reflects a deep cultural divide, or whether cultures might eventually reach agreement on the issue in question. Thanks to Bonnie Steinbock for helping to clarify this point.

17. Interestingly, one study noted that European Americans, the group that is assumed to be in favor of full disclosure in hopes of facilitating an autonomous decision, had only a 63-percent response in favor of telling a patient about a diagnosis of metastatic cancer (Marshall et al. 1998). This seems quite low given that European Americans are often perceived as viewing the patient as an individual who desires information in order to facilitate an autonomous treatment decision.

18. At issue here is the idea that she would be deprived of the fact that such time is quite limited.

19. There is a risk that what is said might not be translated accurately. This lack of accuracy may be intentional, as in the case of Mrs. Chen, or unintentional due, for example, to a translator's lack of understanding of medical terminology. As a general rule, it is best not to use family members as translators (especially in cases where sexual issues are involved).

20. If a family member had not been used as a translator in this case, then Mrs. Chen would most likely have been told about her diagnosis much earlier. To avoid a situation in which a patient is told of a diagnosis against her wishes, healthcare practitioners need to begin such discussions by asking how much information (if any) the patient wants to be given about her condition. If the patient does want information about her condition, the healthcare practitioner needs to be methodical in delivering the information, making sure to stop frequently to allow the patient ample opportunity to ask questions and request not to get any further information (at least for the time being) if she so chooses.

21. For an exemplary method of getting across information to a patient in a manner appropriate to the individual patient, see Freedman, "Offering Truth: One Ethical Approach to the Uninformed Cancer Patient" (2003).

22. Even though autonomy, broadly construed, still seems to be the trumping value (as is common to Western medicine), it does not follow that healthcare practitioners are not being culturally sensitive. Cultural sensitivity calls not for disavowing autonomy as a primary value in the decision-making process, but rather, being open to a variety of interpretations and manifestations of autonomy, *in addition to* being open to ranking autonomy as lower in priority than other values.

23. An interesting example of where an understanding of common cultural practices does not reflect what individual members of that particular culture want for themselves is noted by Tamura (2006). Specifically, recent data in a Japanese poll revealed that a majority of individuals preferred to know the truth about diagnosis, even when it was grim. "In 2000, one of the biggest newspaper companies in Japan conducted a large-scale survey of the general population . . . [which] found that 76% of people said they would want to be told if they had cancer, but only 37% thought that they should tell another family member when that individual was diagnosed

with cancer" (Tamura 2006). Thus, while sensitivity to different cultures and the values therein may entail some acquaintance with cultural practices, at the individual level, other interests may not align with common cultural practice.

24. To be sure, different guidelines apply when dealing with a pediatric population.

25. Most state laws regarding medical consent function to protect physicians from charges of "battery." Left open by the law in most cases is the moral question of how to respect adequately a patient's autonomy.

26. As a general rule, information ought to be offered as least every couple of days and more often if there is a change in or new information regarding the patient's condition.

27. One may contend that it is culturally biased to insist on putting the patient in a position to choose how informed she wants to be. However, as noted earlier in the chapter, a culturally sensitive practitioner, while striving to understand and respect the values and beliefs of other cultures, is operating within the confines of American law. As such, certain guidelines must be followed. In this case, practitioners need to obtain informed consent (or refusal), hopefully, in a manner that accords with or is least offensive to the patient.

28. In Japan, for example, advance directives do not have any legal standing.

29. Though the outcome for members of certain populations might be the same—namely, a refusal to engage in advance care planning or fill out an advance directive—the reasons underlying such decisions vary widely. For instance, research indicates that African Americans might come to this conclusion based on a distrust of the medical system, while Navajos might reach the same conclusion for the reasons mentioned above.

30. Navajo culture is not alone in its lack of acceptance when it comes to advance care planning. Chinese culture holds that in talking about illness and disease, one is inviting such maladies to befall one.

31. This inclusive approach, if favored by the patient, would be an acceptable (if not favorable) approach in Western cultures as well.

32. A useful source of information on cross-cultural health care is a computer-based information system developed by two Minnesota hospitals: see Meyer, *Medicine's Melting Pot*, 1996, as cited in Setness (1998).

33. Thanks to Kerry Bowman for making this point clear.

WORKS CITED

American Medical Student Association. 2005. *Cultural competency in medicine.* http://www/amsa.org/programs/gpit/cultural.cfm (accessed December 21, 2005).

Berger, J. T. 1998. Culture and ethnicity in clinical care. *Archives of Internal Medicine* 158:2085–90.

Blackhall, L. J., G. Frank, S. Murphy, and V. Michel. 2001. Bioethics in a different tongue: The case of truth-telling. *Journal of Urban Health* 78 (1): 59–67.

Bowman, K. In press. *Understanding and respecting cultural differences in end-of-life care.*

CBC. 2006. *CBC news online.* www.cbc.ca/story/science/national/2006/03/01/ translate-health060301.html (accessed June 2, 2006).

Engel, G. L. 1977. The need for a new medical model: A challenge for biomedicine. *Science* 196 (4286): 129–36.

Flores, G., J. Rabke-Verani, W. Pine, and A. Sabharwal. 2002. The importance of cultural and linguistic issues in the emergency care of children. *Pediatric Emergency Care* 18 (4): 271–84.

Freedman, B. 2003. Offering truth: One ethical approach to the uninformed cancer patient. In *Ethical issues in modern medicine,* ed. by B. Steinbock, J. D. Arras, and A. J. London, 76–82. New York: McGraw-Hill.

Galanti, G. 2004. *Caring for patients from different cultures.* 3rd ed. Philadelphia: University of Pennsylvania Press.

Haffner, L. 1992. Translation is not enough. *The Western Journal of Medicine* 157 (3): 255.

Hern, H. E., Jr., B. A. Koenig, L. J. Moore, and P. A. Marshall. 1998. The difference that culture can make in end-of-life decision making. *Cambridge Quarterly of Healthcare Ethics* 7:27–40.

Hester, D. M. 2001. *Community as healing: Pragmatist ethics in medical encounters.* Lanham, MD: Rowman & Littlefield.

Jecker, N. S., J. A. Carrese, and R. A. Pearlman. 1995. Caring for patients in cross cultural settings. *Hastings Center Report* 25 (6): 6–14.

Juckett, G. 2005. Cross-cultural medicine. *American Family Physician* 72 (11): 2267–74.

Kekes, J. 1996. *The morality of pluralism.* Princeton, NJ: Princeton University Press.

Klessig, J. 1992. The effect of values and culture on life-support decisions. *The Western Journal of Medicine* 157 (3): 316.

Macklin, R. 2006. Ethical relativism in a multicultural society. In *Biomedical ethics,* 6th ed., edited by T. A. Mappes and D. Degrazia, 118–27. New York: McGraw-Hill.

Marshall, P. A., B. A. Koenig, D. M. Barnes, and A. J. Davis. 1998. Multiculturalism, bioethics, and end-of-life care: Case narratives of Latino cancer patients. In *Health care ethics: Critical issues for the 21st century,* edited by J. F. Monagle and D. C. Thomasma, 421–31. Sudbury: Jones and Bartlett.

Muller, J. H., and B. Desmond. 1992. Ethical dilemmas in a cross-cultural context: A Chinese example. *The Western Journal of Medicine* 157 (3): 323.

Parens, E. 1998. What differences make a difference? *Cambridge Quarterly of Healthcare Ethics* 7:1–6.

Pelligrino, E. 1979. The anatomy of clinical judgments: Some notes on right reason and right action. In *Clinical judgment: A critical appraisal,* ed. H. T. Engelhardt, S. F. Spicker, and B. Towers, 169–94. Dordrecht: Reidel.

Powell, T. 2006. Culture and communication: Medical disclosure in Japan and the U.S. *The American Journal of Bioethics* 6 (1): 18–20.

Ramsey, P. 1970. *The patient as a person.* New Haven, CT: Yale University Press.

Rawls, J. 1971. *A theory of justice.* Cambridge: The Belknap Press of Harvard University Press.

Rosenblat, H., and P. Hong. 1989. Coin rolling misdiagnosed as child abuse. *Canadian Medical Association Journal* 140:417.

Setness, P. A. 1998. Culturally competent healthcare: Meeting challenges can improve outcomes and enrich patient care. *Postgraduate Medicine Online* 103 (2): 13.

Steinbock, B., J. D. Arras, and A. J. London, eds. 2003. *Ethical issues in modern medicine*. New York: McGraw-Hill.

Tamura, C. 2006. The family-facilitated approach could be dangerous if there is pressure by family dynamics. *The American Journal of Bioethics* 6 (1): 16–18.

Valle, R. 2001. Cultural assessment in bioethical advocacy—Toward cultural competency in bioethical practice. *Bioethics Forum* 17 (1): 15–26.

7

Religious Values and Medical Decision Making

Toby L. Schonfeld

KEY POINTS

1. Describe the ways that a patient's religious or spiritual values influence medical decision making.
2. Explain why discussions of religious or spiritual issues should not be automatically delegated to Pastoral Care or other specialty services.
3. List at least three areas of health care where religious values commonly prescribe or proscribe particular actions.
4. Articulate strategies for negotiation with patients who refuse care on religious grounds or who make unorthodox treatment requests or decisions.

Case 1: Refusal of Blood Transfusion

G. B. is a six-year-old African American boy with known sickle cell disease. He presented with a two-day history of fatigue, poor appetite, and pallor, and a six-hour history of rapid and loud breathing. He lived with his mother and two unmarried aunts, all of whom were Jehovah's Witnesses.

On examination, G. B. was lethargic, tachycardic, tachypneic, and in moderate distress. Systolic BP was low, and perfusion was decreased. Tests showed a mildly elevated white blood cell count and a very low hemoglobin of 3 gm/dl with a markedly decreased reticulocyte count at 0.1 percent. A chest x-ray showed a significantly enlarged heart and diffuse pulmonary edema. Oxygen saturation improved

---

with the administration of oxygen, but fell again after fluids were given for the low blood pressure.

It was considered likely that G. B. was in high-output cardiac failure secondary to severe anemia, probably as a result of an aplastic crisis. His mother, supported by her sister and church elders, refused red blood cell transfusion, suggesting instead treatment with erythropoietin. A court order was obtained, and G. B. was transfused and recovered uneventfully. (Gordon)

Most ethics committee members are familiar with cases like G. B.'s described above, where a family's religious commitments influence the decision it will make about the course of treatment for themselves or a loved one. In the particular case of Jehovah's Witnesses refusing blood or blood products, the situation has been common enough to generate well-known legal precedents and relatively "settled" moral opinion. On the one hand, adult Jehovah's Witnesses, just like adults without those particular religious beliefs, may refuse even life-sustaining care as long as that adult has decisional capacity and can demonstrate that he or she fully understands the consequences of this decision (Furrow et al. 2000).

However, the situation differs with regard to minors (Linnard-Palmer and Kools 2004). The courts have consistently held (Furrow et al. 2000) that insofar as minors lack the life experience and cognitive development that enables them to weigh these decisions among other goals, values, and priorities, and to integrate them with a coherent concept of future, minors are not permitted to make these decisions. Instead, parents or guardians who presumably *do* possess these characteristics make the decisions that they consider to be in the "best interests" of the minor. Conflict arises when these decision makers and the healthcare team disagree about precisely what is in the minor's best interests. The religious commitments of Jehovah's Witnesses, like G. B.'s family, require them to refuse blood or blood products on behalf of the minor, even when such intervention is required to save the minor's life. Many healthcare providers find themselves at odds with such decisions, and as a result, have pursued legal action to compel the minors to undergo treatment. Because blood transfusions in many[1] cases represent short-term, temporary, low-risk interventions to which most "reasonable" parents would consent, parental objection about the minor receiving blood or blood products is overridden in the interest of providing for the minor's "best interests" (Furrow et al. 2000).

The case of Jehovah's Witnesses and blood products represents one instance of religious values influencing medical decision making. And while it is important to be aware of this example in order to craft institutional policies or clinical procedures regarding transfusions, committee members would be remiss to think that the "settled" nature of these cases removes any of the moral or emotional angst from the clinical situation. What is at stake in the case of Jehovah's Witnesses is eternal salvation—a consequence to be weighed seriously, to say the least. And while not all examples of religion in health care surround such dire concepts, they all relate to fundamental questions of meaning and how individuals see themselves and their relationship to the world. Ethics committee members and other healthcare professionals would do well to consider religious values and spiritual commitments as instances of attempts to live meaningful lives.

In this chapter, we will focus on not only cases of conflict in health care but also how issues of religion and spirituality permeate the culture of medicine and the lives of the patients for whom we care. The chapter includes information regarding *who* should address these issues as well as *how* they should be approached. Beyond these explicit considerations, committee members are further encouraged to reflect on their own religious or spiritual commitments and how these values affect the perspective they offer to a case consultation.

VALUES: FOUNDATIONS AND FAITH

A typical ethics consultation will begin with a conversation: often it is a conversation between the patient, family members, and caregivers where the group explores the current situation and context and plans a course of action. In order to be a truly successful consultation, however, the consultant needs to elicit the values that underlie the positions of the various parties to the decision. These values ground an individual's or group's position, and it is interest in or fidelity to these values, when confronted by other values, that often results in conflict in the health care setting. Consider the following example:

Case 2: Quality vs. Quantity of Life

A. R., a twenty-nine-year-old woman with two small children, is diagnosed with locally advanced pancreatic cancer. With aggressive therapy, her chance for one-year survival is 20 percent and her chance for five-year survival is 2 percent. The average survival after diagnosis is eight to nine months. Her physicians propose a course of radiation and chemotherapy using an experimental protocol. The side effects include profound fatigue and nausea, in addition to the pain of the cancer itself. Her husband wants her to proceed. She wonders whether it would be better to forgo treatment and emphasize pain management in the hope that her remaining time with the family will be of better quality. (Anderson 2005)

Recognizing that the definitive prognosis for patients with this pancreatic cancer is limited, the physicians recommend a course of treatment for Ms. R. based on the potential of this therapy to extend her life. Ms. R's husband, who presumably does not want to lose her, concurs with this choice. Yet Ms. R herself, also cognizant of her poor prognosis, considers other goals: the desire to maximize her ability to participate in the activities of her friends and family before she dies. These apparently divergent goals (crudely stated here in terms of quantity versus quality) derive from fundamentally different values, that is, from fundamentally different notions about what ought to be protected and supported when making difficult decisions.

In a case such as this one, often consensus is not far off. What is required is for someone to illuminate the different values and goals at play and to facilitate discussion about how to reconcile these notions. Ethics committee consultations can provide just this kind of illumination. In this case, once the medical team understands that the patient values quality over longevity, the team may have suggestions for other care plans that better accommodate these goals.

Suppose, however, that A. R. was a faithful Roman Catholic. How would this have changed the discussion regarding A. R.'s care plan? For one thing, Ms. R. (and perhaps her family) would likely have considered how the various treatment alternatives integrated with or furthered her commitment to church doctrine. She may also have considered whether there were any religious principles that helped guide her decision-making process. She may have appealed to precedents in church history for analogous cases. For assistance with these matters, Ms. R. may have contacted her parish priest or requested the assistance of a hospital chaplain or member of the Pastoral Care department for help in working through these theological issues. Regardless of the approach or the possible expansion of the care team to address Ms. R.'s concerns, one thing is clear: for some patients, religious values will have significant weight in the decision-making process.

This fact, however, raises an important question, especially from the perspective of the care team: Are religious values somehow different in kind from other sorts of values? There can be little doubt that they are treated differently both by those who hold them and those who encounter them in others. One might argue that it is because religious values speak to internal matters and are decidedly universal and ultimate. Of course, for those whose loyalties lie in providing optimal medical care, their values function in what seems to be enduringly powerful ways as well. Consider a few of the more traditional values that infuse health care: honesty, competence, compassion, relief from suffering. These values form the core of practice in medicine, where providers incorporate these commonly held values into the routine care they offer to patients (Pellegrino 1979). We can see that these medically "ultimate" values may contrast with those that are religiously based, such as faith and trust in God to perform miracles, the healing power of prayer, or the virtue of suffering.

Alternatively, one might argue that the reason we treat religious values differently is because they are not universally held; for example, experiencing suffering to become more Christlike is certainly not a value for Jews or Hindus. And yet when one considers the history of value development in medicine, one quickly sees that many of the values we currently hold in high regard were not so viewed a short time ago (consider "honesty" and cancer diagnoses in the 1950s). Furthermore, different cultures and families are likely to either have a different core set of values or place different emphases on commonly held values. For some Asian families, the notion of an autonomous individual may be anathema; instead, recognizing one's role in the family unit requires a reconceptualization of consent in terms of communal responsibility.

In one way, we treat the issue of religious considerations in a manner consistent with the way that we treat other "specialties" in medicine: we use consulting services. When the kidneys become implicated in the disease process, we consult the nephrology team. When the patient will require rehabilitation after a procedure, we consult with physical and occupational therapists. So, in a parallel manner, when the patient requires help resolving spiritual issues or with questions of faith, we consult with Pastoral Care or other spiritual experts.

At first blush, this seems like a perfectly reasonable course of action: when we need someone with different expertise, we call in a specialist. However, upon deeper reflection, this practice, if taken as the immediate and standard response to the expression of religious interests by patients, becomes suspect. In no other situation in health care do we "turf" the discussion of *values* to others . . . unless we find those values suspect. For example, when a patient expresses a desire to forgo a routine, but lifesaving, intervention in favor of a slow and painful death, we question the patient's decisional capacity and call for a psychiatric consult. When a parent or guardian demonstrates fidelity to values that the healthcare team judges are not in the minor's best interests, the team may pursue a court order to appoint a third-party guardian to make decisions—presumably "better" decisions—for the minor. In both cases, the team hopes that the consultants will override the values in question to bring them more in line with those of the healthcare team.

A parallel situation may arise with referrals to Pastoral Care. In many cases, even if this was not the intended effect of a Pastoral Care consult, the upshot is the same: we want the patients to stop the "God talk" and come to their senses about treatment. This approach is neither effective nor desirable, as it has the effect of parsing the patient into separate realms of being—one medical, the other spiritual—and thus separating the patient from a primary source of support. In the next section, we will discuss why it is important to consider religious values and spiritual concerns as a routine part of patient care, and why the patient's primary healthcare provider is the best person to assess these needs.

WHO SHOULD HAVE THESE DISCUSSIONS AND WHY

There are some very practical reasons why only[2] referring patients to clergy or Pastoral Care may not be in their best interests. For one thing, just like with any other consultation service, there may be a significant wait before a representative can visit the patient, as well as significant system pressures that present barriers to consultation (Feudtner et al. 2003). Alternatively, and more important, patients might feel as though they are being compartmentalized, that only some of their concerns are worthy of discussion by the primary providers, and the rest of the conversation must be handled by others. In the meantime, any fear or anxiety the patient feels about his or her medical situation may be prolonged. As Katherine A. Brown-Saltzman comments:

> These are times when our accessibility to the patient will provide opportunities to tend the spirit and to care for the whole person in his or her precious complexity. We have an open door to intimacy and connection if we are respectful and trustworthy. And then, if we begin where the patient is, if we can be present, we have . . . signposts that can guide and heal. (Brown-Saltzman 1994)

Here, Brown-Saltzman (1994) notes the fundamental connection that already exists between the patient and the provider. This relationship provides the "open door to intimacy" necessary to begin the conversation about religious values or spiritual commitments. Any consultant, no matter how qualified, will most often have to establish a relationship with the patient before it will become a safe space for these kinds of considerations. Thus, using consultants as "first line" providers for spiritual considerations is an inefficient way to discover the patient's deepest concerns about his or her care or situation. Instead, one should recognize that the uniquely intimate characteristic of physician-patient relationships is a useful tool in opening dialogue on religious matters related to healthcare.

However, whether talking about the practices of attending physicians or, should it get that far, ethics committee members, there remains the issue of qualifications on religious matters. Most physicians are not clergy, and many ethics committee members find religious concerns uncomfortable. Thus, why should such persons muck around in these difficult matters when chaplains are available? Certainly it seems like those with experience engaging in discussions of ultimate meaning and religious beliefs are the best equipped to help patients work through these issues. In some respects, this is true for those who have particular questions about how a certain intervention or plan of care is viewed in a specific religious tradition. For example, if a patient questions whether a do-not-resuscitate order (DNR) is sanctioned by Judaism, asking a rabbi is a good course of action. However, patients' concerns are often more general than this. Even when they couch it in religious language, frequently, patients simply are expressing the need for a willing ear to listen to their hopes and fears about their treatment (Curlin and Hall 2005; Handzo and Koenig

2004; Curlin et al. 2005). As Brown-Saltzman notes, "[p]atients ask in the crisis of the moment, in their anxiousness and despair; they are not hoping to receive definitive answers but rather are asking us to help make sense of their plight and to help find ways to hope, to live, and sometimes to die" (Brown-Saltzman 1994).

Note that depending on how one views such a conversation, either none of us has particular expertise in these areas, or else we all do. In his books *The Measure of Our Days* (1997) and *The Anatomy of Hope* (2004), Jerome Groopman makes the case that we all have the power to tend to the spirit and help our patients maintain hope regardless of the clinical picture. Furthermore, one could argue that to fail to provide for this conversation with patients is to fail to complete a basic component of care for the patient (Curlin et al. 2005; Puchalski 2001), especially given the evidence that states that patients want their providers to inquire into their spiritual needs (Kliewer 2004; Ehman et al. 1999; LaPierre 1994). Therefore, the risk of failing to engage the patient in these conversations is the risk of abandonment.

Furthermore, there are positive benefits that can result from the integration of religion and health care (Butler et al. 2003). Certainly spiritual commitments to a force greater than oneself can help a patient transcend the difficulties of health problems and can work together with traditional medicine toward overall healing (Trier and Shupe 1991; Duckro and Magaletta 1994). The social nature of religious communities can contribute not only important psychological or emotional support for patients, but can in fact alter behavior as well. For example, one study demonstrated that involvement in a religious community was associated with a low-fat diet (Hart et al. 2004).

One barrier to having conversations about religion in health care comes when providers or ethics consultants are uncomfortable because they do not know how to ask the questions (Ehman et al. 1999) or because they are afraid of offending patients who may believe differently than the providers themselves (Monroe et al. 2003). This fear comes from a recognition of religious and spiritual diversity and an acknowledgment that one's own religious beliefs or practices come second to the needs of the patient. When a patient asks a provider to pray with—or for—her, the provider may not know how to respond without giving offense (either by praying in a manner that would offend the patient or by refusing to pray at all). This is where the importance of dialogue and a relationship come in. One response to the question "Will you pray for me?" is "What would you like me to pray for?" The answer to this question can shed some light onto the patient's spiritual needs and how best to meet them. If the provider focuses on listening rather than talking, on being a nonanxious presence with whom patients feel safe describing their fears, offense is unlikely to occur.

A more common barrier, however, is the provider or ethics consultant who is uncomfortable engaging in these conversations because he or she has difficulty coming to terms with questions of ultimate meaning in his or her own life. Helping a parent understand the death of a child or working through the challenges with a newly paralyzed patient may cause the provider to question his or her own belief system and source of meaning. For that reason, it is crucial that providers and ethics committee members alike make the time to reflect on their own religious beliefs and sources of spiritual support on a regular basis. Only by taking account of our own sources of meaning will we be effective companions for our patients as they struggle through their journeys.

Of course, sometimes religious values are not addressed with patients simply because they do not arise in the conversation. For some people of faith, health care is a separate realm and so medical decisions, especially less significant ones, do not require spiritual consultation. And many other patients, certainly, will not be people of faith, and for them such conversations are moot . . . or are they?

I would argue that even for those patients who do not express fidelity to a particular religious creed or make any reference to faith-based considerations, issues of *spirituality* are nonetheless relevant. The terms "religion" and "spirituality" are used in many different ways in both clinical contexts and the literature, but one thing remains clear: when faced with a difficult or unexpected diagnosis, or when life-altering decisions are pending, many individuals are thrown into crises of meaning that require the consideration of questions of ultimate import (O'Neill and Kenny 1998). This situation is often termed a "crisis of faith," and as such typically refers only to those individuals who *have* a particular religious faith to question. Yet all of us, religious or not, have a particular understanding of our place in the world and as beings who relate in some way to others. Knowing "what it all means" is by no means solely the domain of religion, and those without formal religious beliefs have needs that go to the heart of living meaningfully in relation to one's environment and communities as well (Baggini and Pym 2005; Hester 2001). Yet we frequently divert such conversations to those with "expertise" in that field. However, as I have already argued, carving out discussions of deep life-significance and meaning (religious or otherwise) from the general discussion of patient preferences and goals does a disservice to the patient and robs the care team of important insight into the patient's system of values.

HOW CAN RELIGIOUS VALUES INTERSECT WITH HEALTH-CARE DECISION MAKING?

Each patient brings his or her own set of special concerns to the healthcare milieu. Emphasizing this fact is an important reminder that healthcare providers must look beyond physiology and biochemistry to include the ways that healthy living gains meaning for individual patients. Religious values (broadly conceived as values of meaningful living) affect the decisional considerations for many patients. Some will be members of organized religious traditions with defined rules about what is and is not permitted for members of their faith. Others will enter the medical realm with personal convictions based on individual spiritual commitments. Regardless, the best way to assess the patient's religious and spiritual needs is to engage in dialogue with patients to discover the nature of their beliefs and how those beliefs might affect treatment decisions.

Even though the nature of religious values always takes on a very specific character when expressed by an individual, it is still useful to look at some general areas of health management and decision making where values based on commitment to certain organized religions may come into play for specific individuals. Below, then, is a list of common considerations regarding religious values, that is, a list of areas in which individuals may have religious commitments that affect the care they are willing to receive. The goal of this section is to familiarize the reader with the kinds of considerations patients with religious commitments may present to the provider. This list is *not* intended to serve as a definitive catalog of faith traditions and their approaches to health care. Consequently, there are several caveats to be offered with this list:

1. The list is neither exhaustive nor exclusive, but simply represents the most commonly discussed intersections of health care and religious values.
2. There is a great deal of variety within each religious tradition, and such considerations lead to the necessity of discussing with the patient where on the continuum he or she falls.
3. Not every member of a religious tradition practices in the same way, so even if you know the house of worship or clergy member to whom the patient has allegiance, it does not follow that you know exactly how that patient will make medical decisions. In the same vein, it is not always clear how an individual's religious commitments will affect medical decision making or the care provided—if at all.
4. Since in several faith traditions, the requirement to preserve life and health trumps other considerations, other religious rules may be overruled in light of what is required for healing.

Therefore, while this list will serve to introduce concepts of religious value and medical decision making, it should by no means be considered a substitute for a meaningful conversation between the provider and the patient. In fact, it is terribly important to avoid the temptation to think that since someone is, for example, Roman Catholic, that it follows that she or he is necessarily against birth control or even abortion. However, such general knowledge about religious precepts can act as a stimulant for conversation by providing enough information to generate useful and meaningful questions in relation to patients and patient families and their goals for medical intervention.

Dietary Restrictions

All other things being equal, the dietary laws that apply to the daily lives of members of certain religions will also apply when these members are sick or hospitalized. The most notable of these restrictions are for Jews and Muslims, who are likely to request vegetarian meals when institutionalized in order to comply with their religious commitments regarding the procurement and preparation of meat. There are other traditions that have less well-known restrictions: groups that will consume no caffeine, for example. A great many hospitals are familiar with these restrictions and often have provisions in their dietary support systems for these purposes (for example, by having kosher meals available for Jews or certified halal meat for Muslims). Alternatively, individuals from within the patient's religious community may bring food to the hospital for the patient. This action is considered a religious obligation for members of several religious traditions.

Certain times of year may pose particular challenges for the observant patient. During Ramadan, Muslims will not consume food or beverage during daylight hours. During Passover, Jews will not eat anything made with a leavening agent. And during Lent, Roman Catholics abstain from meat on Fridays. Because these events follow lunar calendars, the dates will not correspond exactly from year to year with the secular calendar. The healthcare provider must rely on the patient to disclose this information, and then be willing to discuss the implications of this observance for his or her treatment regimen.

There are some who worry that the religious prohibitions on ingesting certain kinds of foods (pork, for example) extend to other products made from these animals: pig valves for hearts or porcine-derived insulin, for example. In at least one religious tradition, the prohibition extends only to those things ingested by mouth. Therefore, products derived from prohibited sources are permitted, although there is a preference for products derived from other sources when available and effective (synthetic insulin, for example).

This is one area where the duty to preserve life and health may take precedence over a religious restriction. The ingestion of prohibited substances, when required to save a life, is often either sanctioned or specifically required by religious authorities. Whether a particular instance of food or beverage intake qualifies under this provision must be negotiated with the patient, family, and often with religious representatives.

Modesty and Personal Space

Certain religious traditions, such as some conservative Christian faiths, Hinduism, Islam, and some forms of Judaism, include provisions for maintaining personal modesty, especially for women. As a result, there is a preference for a provider who is the same sex as the patient if possible. Additionally, while ensuring that a patient's body is appropriately covered is an important feature of respect for patients, it takes on particular importance in these contexts. Considerations of modesty are sometimes related to notions of bodily integrity, which has implications for the care of the body regarding surgery or after death (see below).

For some religious traditions, physically touching someone can have negative connotations (for positive aspects of touching, see below). Generally, touching that is necessary for an intervention to preserve the life or health of an individual is sanctioned; however, additional touching may raise concerns. For a Muslim man, being touched by a woman, especially a non-Muslim woman, after he has performed the ablutions necessary for prayer is problematic. Similar problems arise when members of other religious traditions are touched by nonmembers, particularly when the patient is near death. These problems are sometimes exacerbated when the touching is done by a member of the opposite sex. As a result, it is wise to inquire about the permissibility of touching with the patient and his or her family.

Pain and Suffering

The extent to which pain and suffering should be alleviated may rest on the patient's religious values. Some traditions find meaning in suffering as a transformative process or as a means to pursuing the understanding that leads to salvation. Some see pain and suffering as a divine punishment for wrongdoing or on account of transgressions in a past life. A few traditions view suffering as not only beneficial but necessary in order to approximate Christ's suffering for His people. However, these attempts to find meaning in suffering may work collaboratively with, rather than instead of, medical interventions geared toward the alleviation of pain and suffering. Some, like Buddhists or Hindus, may reject pain medication that dulls the senses and interferes with their ability to be "mindful" of their situation or actively involved in the dying process. Other traditions, by contrast, regard suffering as unnecessary and undesirable and something to be overcome at all costs.

These differences, while marked, are not at all obvious, and may vary from location to location. Given that these values may significantly impact the treatment alternatives that a patient and his or her family may consider, it is incumbent upon the provider to assess for the patient's understanding of the value or disvalue of pain and suffering.

Even for those traditions that sanction the relief of pain and suffering, there may be limits. In chronic conditions where pain is significant, adequate pain relief may come with the added element of unconsciousness or decreased respiration. The possibility of pain management hastening death is problematic for some religious traditions, and as a result, patients and families may set boundaries for what is or is not acceptable regarding pain relief. Providers are also often encouraged to seek nonpharmacological remedies for pain. Additionally, psychological comforts, such as the laying on of hands, may have spiritual significance as well as provide emotional support for patients and families.

Medications

As mentioned previously, the dietary prohibitions against certain animal products may extend to anything ingested orally. A patient may ask about the origins of a particular product in order to ascertain its permissibility according to his or her religious values. One religious tradition in particular, Seventh Day Adventists, will not take any over-the-counter medication.

A patient may also have religious objections to using medications on other grounds. Some patients refuse routine vaccinations for their children on the grounds that the serum was developed through immoral means. Typically, the patients for whom this is a concern will be well-versed in these areas and come prepared to discuss these values and their implication with the healthcare provider. Given that these considerations have import for public health, some professional organizations have taken positions against this practice. Even these groups, however, recommend respecting parents' refusal "after adequate discussion . . . unless the child is put at significant risk of serious harm" (Diekema and the Committee on Bioethics 2005).

Childbearing

Rituals surrounding pregnancy and birth are varied and plentiful, as many religious traditions have some way to sanctify bringing new life into the world. Religious considerations factor into the equation throughout the continuum of conception to birth.

Contraception

Restrictions on contraceptive measures are well known for some religious traditions. Roman Catholics, for example, seek to make every procreative act open to the possibility of conception (all things being equal). As a result, contraceptive measures are generally rejected. Similarly, Orthodox Jews understand the religious precept to "be fruitful and multiply" to encourage a couple to welcome any product of a procreative act. In both of these cases, however, some exceptions have been made for the health—both physical and psychological—of the mother. Some forms of birth control are more palatable to observant individuals than others based on other religious values. In the case of contraception, as with many decisions in health care, decision making is a balancing act of competing interests and conflicting commitments. The way in which such a weighing of options is resolved will likely differ case by case.

Conception

In an era when many individuals seek assistance in conceiving a child, the once private realm of conception has entered the public domain. As a result, healthcare providers should be aware of religious values that influence notions of infertility and assisted reproduction. In no religious tradition is it required to seek reproductive assistance for infertility, but it is permitted in many. For some traditions, especially those with an emphasis on procreation, most currently available forms of assisted reproductive technologies are sanctioned. For others, religious values may impose some limits on a couple, relating to the ways in which the gametes are retrieved and the method and location of their joining. These limits may either prohibit certain forms of assisted reproduction altogether, or they may require an alteration in the customary procedure for procuring the components of conception. Regardless, an increased sensitivity to the needs of patients both to adhere to their religious commitments and to have a child is warranted.

Prenatal Genetic Counseling

The purpose of prenatal genetic counseling is to obtain additional information about a pregnancy and about the condition of the fetus. Whether such counseling is permitted by various religions depends on (1) how the information is obtained, and (2) the purpose for which the information is requested. For those traditions that staunchly oppose pregnancy termination for any reason, there may be prohibitions against such counseling with the understanding that this additional information may lead couples to seek termination services. Other traditions, even those who oppose pregnancy termination, may sanction such counseling as a way for parents to prepare, both physically and psychologically, for a child with special needs.

Birth

Rather than requiring healthcare providers to perform an action, birth rituals often require the healthcare providers to *refrain from* performing an action that is part of standard care. For example, because of Jews' desire to have their male children circumcised in a religious ceremony outside the hospital, parents will request that their provider not perform the routine circumcision that is otherwise part of standard postnatal care. In other traditions, like the Hmong, the placenta has religious significance, and parents may request that the placenta not be discarded with other extraneous birth products but rather returned to them for sacred burial. Given the idiosyncratic nature of these values, healthcare providers should simply be open to these discussions and accommodating whenever possible.

Pregnancy Termination

Religious values are often brought to bear on the status of the developing fetus and the implications for pregnancy termination. Many, but not all, traditions sanction the termination of a pregnancy whose continuation threatens the life of the mother. This position is defended in a myriad of ways, including through the traditionally Catholic notion of the Doctrine of Double Effect[3] and through the rabbinic view that in such circumstances the fetus is a *rodef*, or pursuer, against whom the woman is required to defend herself. For some traditions, the understanding of the moral standing of the fetus is a developmental one, where the closer to viability, the more moral weight is attached to the fetus.

While many religious traditions have guidelines regarding the acceptability of pregnancy termination, others do not. Patients themselves may be misinformed about their tradition's stance on the issue and may instead be influenced by the divisive rhetoric of popular culture. As a result, inquiring into the patient's spiritual concerns regarding pregnancy termination may engender contacting additional resources for assistance in facilitating the conversation.

Donor Organs or Tissues

All major (recognized) organized religions permit cadaveric organ or tissue donation. In fact, some religious traditions require such donation on the grounds that they serve to preserve the life of another individual. Even those religions with resurrection theologies do not prohibit the donation of organs or tissues. These faiths hold that either (1) one's organs or tissues will not be needed at the time of resurrection, as our existence will be otherworldly, or (2) if one does need particular organs or tissues, God will restore them just as He restored our life force.

Despite the general permissiveness of religious traditions regarding organ and tissue donation, many families are unaware of the official stance of their tradition's governing body and, as a result, question these teachings at the point of decision. Most organ recovery personnel are well-versed in these religious teachings and can help a family work through these issues. Additionally, considering these issues in advance, either in conjunction with the creation of an advance directive or when obtaining a driver's license, can help patients and families navigate this terrain before an emotionally complex situation arises.

Mechanical Ventilation

The ability to sustain ventilation mechanically presented a challenge to religious traditions that historically viewed the cessation of heartbeat and respiration as indicators of death. As a result, the transition to a brain-centered definition of death caused religious leaders to consider what this would mean for members of their community. Some traditions, such as Roman Catholicism, have applied the ordinary/extraordinary distinction to technologies such as these. That is, we are morally required to provide care that the patient or his or her family judges has a reasonable hope of benefit and is not unduly burdensome. In some cases, such as mechanical ventilation during or after surgery or for temporary purposes, mechanical ventilation clearly falls into the "ordinary" category. In other, more long-term cases, its use may indeed be, in the judgment of the patient or his or her family, disproportionately burdensome. In that case, the technology may be removed.

Often, the move to mechanical ventilation, especially long-term, engenders a conversation about the goals of care, specifically regarding quality and quantity of life. These concepts have moral significance in many religious traditions. Islam, for example, values good works and service to God: purposes that can only be exercised if a certain quality of life is maintained. This understanding leads to the position that mechanical ventilation as a temporary measure to restore someone to health or functioning is permissible. However, mechanical ventilation that simply prolongs a person's life without improving his or her ability to fulfill life's purpose would not be sanctioned in Islam.

Artificial Nutrition or Hydration

Some of the most stark differences between religious traditions can be seen in the discussion of the permissibility of starting and, more important, stopping, artificial nutrition and hydration. The (im)permissibility of withholding artificial nutrition and hydration rests on a fundamental distinction in how this technology is viewed. Those religious traditions that view artificial nutrition and hydration as basic sustenance and analogous to food or water that is normally taken by mouth are much less likely to sanction discontinuation of this care for patients. Those traditions that view artificial nutrition and hydration as a form of medicine or mechanical intervention, similar to other interventions like mechanical ventilation, may view the removal of this care acceptable on the grounds that interventions that are not improving the patient's condition may be stopped or withheld. Some traditions maintain a moral distinction between withholding and withdrawing care, which impacts medical decision making.

End-of-Life Issues

Appropriate care for the dying presupposes that we can identify when a patient has reached this point—something that is not always medically possible. Regardless, religious values may become particularly salient at such times.

Special Practices

Roman Catholics and some other Christian traditions may desire the sacrament of Anointing of the Sick. Formerly known as "Last Rites," this ritual has more recently been offered not just to those who are dying, but rather to anyone suffering a grave illness. It is thought both that the sacrament itself has healing powers and that spiritual conviction can be strengthened as the body weakens. Some traditions will require or request baptism, especially for a newborn or child, at the time of death, and many hospital chaplains have the ability and authority to provide this service for patients and their families. Additionally, some patients may prefer to be surrounded by members of their faith community at the time of death. These individuals may read from Scripture, pray, or meditate with and for the patient.

Care for Dying Patients

Some traditions establish the permissibility of actions based on intent, as was discussed previously in relation to the Doctrine of Double Effect. Another example comes from the Anglican tradition, where there is a distinction between those actions that intend care for the dying (through the palliation of symptoms), as compared with those actions whose intent is to actively intend death. A related distinction can be found in Judaism. There, one is not required to provide care that prolongs the dying process. Some sanction the removal of mechanical ventilation in certain circumstances according to this principle. However, one is prohibited from engaging in action that hastens a person's death. Therefore, pain medication that decreases respiration and may hasten death, even though all that is intended is relief from suffering, is not permissible. Finally, not all religious traditions value autonomy equally; end-of-life decisions may relate to family or community concerns as well.

Care for the Body after Death

Many religious traditions have rituals and practices regarding the care for the body after death. Some traditions, like Judaism, reject autopsies unless absolutely required for medical reasons or unless they are required by law. Many faith communities have their own systems for preparing the body for burial. Some require that whenever possible, the body only be touched by members of the faith community. However, if no one is available in the hospital, for example, then hospital personnel may remove tubes, close the eyes of the body, and so forth, until a member of the faith community arrives. Many traditions, such as Islam and Judaism, require the burial of the body with all possible haste. Cremation is prohibited by certain faiths—Judaism and Islam, for example—but is desired by others, like Buddhism, Sikhism, and Hinduism.

UNORTHODOX REQUESTS AND REFUSALS OF CARE

So far, we have discussed how religious values may come into play in the medical arena, as well as reasons why healthcare providers are well situated to have these discussions with patients. While patients need not be members of mainstream religious organizations—or, in fact, adherents of organized religion at all—in order for their religious or spiritual concerns to impact medical decision making, such affiliation does provide some comfort. For one thing, members of recognized religious movements are more likely to be involved with a community of believers who can lend important emotional and spiritual support during times of illness. Additionally, a recognized power structure makes the path toward resources clearer: an established hierarchy provides a mechanism for knowing whom to contact when there are theological questions about a proposed medical intervention. Finally, there is comfort in the familiar: a patient who professes she is a Hindu is likely to receive the benefit of the doubt even if we are unsure as to what those beliefs imply in the medical arena.

Yet there are those patient presentations that challenge our customary notions of belief and that test our limits of accommodation. A patient who refuses lifesaving care on the grounds that, say, the Wizard of Oz will restore her to functioning might reasonably have her decisional capacity called into question. Yet what makes these claims different in kind from those who, for example, refuse blood transfusions on the basis of scriptural interpretation? Why do we accept one choice as legitimate but reject the other as "crazy?"

As Byron Chell points out in his discussion of competency, this distinction cannot simply rest on the concept of irrationality (Chell 1998). After all, even—or perhaps especially—deeply held mainstream religious conviction is, strictly speaking, "irrational" with its faith in truths that are by their very nature unprovable. Understood in this way, it will not work to say that the Jehovah's Witness is "rational" and the Oz devotee is not. Instead, what cases like this turn on are nothing more than what Chell (1998) calls our "common religious experience." Those beliefs and belief systems that fall within this realm gain our respect, and those that fall outside of it do not. Chell (1998) points out that the courts have used similar guidelines to decide what counts as a "religion," whose free exercise is constitutionally protected.

Of course, decisional capacity requires more than simply that an individual's beliefs fall within our common religious experience. As with any capacity determination, the patient must demonstrate that she understands the consequences of the decision she is making and that it falls within her life plan and value system. *Respect for religious beliefs or values is not the same as sanctioning psychological denial.* For example, a patient's family might hold the religious value that artificial nutrition and hydration are forms of basic sustenance and cannot be discontinued from a patient in, say, a persistent vegetative state. However, this belief is different and separate from the belief that the patient could be fed orally if providers just tried a bit harder. It is incumbent upon health care providers to engage in frequent dialogue with a patient or family to help them come to terms with the medical reality of the situation. Only then can religious values be applied to the benefit of the patient.

What about those patients whose religious beliefs fall within the realm of common experience, and yet whose individual actions still challenge providers? There is a continuum of such concerns, ranging from the Christian Scientist who, as a rule, rejects all form of Western medical care, to those individual members of religious communities who rely on faith healing instead of, or in addition to, traditional medical care. Consider the following case:

Case 3: Illness as Divine Retribution

Emma Chapman, a sixty-two-year-old black woman, was admitted to the coronary care unit because she had continued episodes of acute chest pain after two heart attacks. Her physician recommended an angiogram with a possible cardiac bypass or angioplasty to follow. Mrs. Chapman refused, saying, "If my faith is strong enough and if it is meant to be, God will cure me." Although Mrs. Chapman never provided any details, she believed she had sinned and her illness was a punishment . . . illnesses from "natural causes: can be treated through nature . . . , but diseases caused by 'sin' can be cured only through God's intervention." (Galanti 1997)

Ms. Chapman's conviction that illness was a punishment for sin clearly demonstrates the spiritual crisis she is experiencing. Calling in resources, such as hospital chaplains or her personal clergy, is an appropriate way to help her work through this crisis. Continuing to engage Ms. Chapman in discussion and partnering with resources such as Pastoral Care will ensure continuity of care and assist the patient in feeling supported as she works through these issues. Until Ms. Chapman is able to make spiritual peace with her situation, it is unlikely that she will be a willing participant in her medical care.

A similar process can be followed when patients and families assert that they are "waiting for a miracle" and therefore refuse medical intervention. The "miracle" language can often be code for several considerations, including but not limited to: (1) patients and families may feel as though engaging in aggressive therapies somehow undermines the power of God to heal and is therefore a wrong choice for the faithful; (2) patients and families may be in denial about the realities of the medical situation and use the miracle terminology as a way of shutting down the conversation; or (3) patients and families may truly understand the medical situation, and yet their spiritual or religious commitments continue to give them hope in spite of long odds. Because these considerations require very different actions on the part of the healthcare team, it will be extremely useful to have the assistance of Pastoral Care in assessing the needs of the patient or family with respect to these particular concerns.

It is important to distinguish those traditions like the Church of Christ Scientist (Christian Science) that rely exclusively on faith healing as a response to infirmity, from those traditions that believe in the restorative powers of prayer as a helpful companion to Western medicine. In fact, many religious traditions have special prayers that are recited to speed healing or to comfort those who are ill. Sometimes these are recited by the patient and sometimes by others in the community on the patient's behalf. The knowledge that others are praying for one can be healing and comforting for the patient. There is, in fact, evidence to suggest that prayer—intercessory or otherwise—may positively affect patient outcomes (Levin 2003; Palmer et al. 2004). Regardless, what is noteworthy here is that individuals who believe in the power of prayer for healing ought not be grouped with those who, for example, rely on the Wizard of Oz for a cure. Instead, it is best to consider prayerful patients as those who have a rich spiritual well from which to draw.

Finally, spiritual commitments that accompany cultural practices novel to the provider may cause some antagonism if not approached properly. In her book *When Doctors Say No* (Rubin 1998), Sue Rubin describes the case of a woman from Southeast Asia whose medical care had reached the point of medical futility (pp. 74–75). Despite this, the patient continued to insist that treatment must continue. This was a problem for the treatment team, who desired to move to comfort care only once the futility determination was made. It was not until much later that, in a detailed conversation, the source of the patient's concern was revealed. According to her spiritual beliefs, if she were to die while the moon was in the current phase, her spirit could not ascend to its resting place. She was merely asking for treatment to be continued for a few extra days out of respect for her spiritual beliefs. Once understood in this way, the patient's request looked reasonable: she understood the situation and its consequences, and was simply asking for a short extension of care to preserve her spiritual integrity. The treatment team was able to comply with this request, and the patient survived until the next phase of the moon.

This case demonstrates the importance of engaging in a conversation with the patient or her family about their spiritual commitments and the ways they may interact with health care. And while the provider did not share this patient's beliefs, respect for those beliefs enabled the parties to reach a satisfactory conclusion together.

One caveat should be offered with regard to respect for religious diversity. Approaching each case with an open mind regarding a patient's spiritual commitments is a good starting point, since the diversity of religious belief and expression may have unexpected applications to medical decision making. However, fidelity to the precepts of religious tolerance does not commit one to relativism. As was evidenced in the example of the Oz devotee, it is not the case that all religious beliefs and practices are, as we sometimes say, created equal. The courts have made these distinctions, for example, in relation to the involvement of children in Native American peyote rituals or as members of snake handling groups. It is also important to distinguish between religious practices and cultural norms, which can be seen in the difference in the history between male and female circumcision.[4] Respect for religious practices cannot, and should not, be done blindly; rather, the provider should seek to educate himself or herself about the context surrounding the patient's refusal or acceptance of care by engaging in dialogue about the patient's religious faith.

CONCLUSION

Providers and ethics committee members should approach issues of religion in health care in much the same way that they approach any sort of value discussion with patients: by asking open-ended questions geared toward identifying the patient's values, goals, and priorities. The way a person orders her life is often reflected in the choices she makes regarding health care, and thus the way to understand these decisions is to consider them in the larger context. Religious values work the same way: commitments outside of the healthcare arena may affect the choices patients make inside the medical realm. Yet only by engaging the patient in conversation about these commitments and what they mean for this patient in particular will the provider know the best way to proceed in the present circumstances. Religious values in health care are not simply about court orders and faith healing; rather, religious values vary greatly in content and form. The application of such values is often nuanced and subtle, and it may require only minor deviations from the provider's routine course of action. Providers should partner with resources such as Pastoral Care, ethics committee members, or community members, rather than delegate the entire dialogue to these individuals. Doing so will enable the provider to maintain the provider-patient relationship while at the same time addressing the patient's religious or spiritual need.

FOR FURTHER REFLECTION

1. How do religious values influence medical decision making?
2. Who should discuss religious commitments with patients?

3. What kinds of religious values might providers expect to encounter?
4. Must providers respect all religious values equally?

NOTES

1. Usually the understanding is that transfusions are a once-and-done (or perhaps twice-and-done) intervention. This is not always the case, however. In 2002, the Canadian press reported on the case of Bethany Hughes, a sixteen-year-old suffering from acute myeloid leukemia. At the time of her death in September 2002, she had undergone thirty-eight blood transfusions against her will and against the wishes of her mother and sisters. For more information about this case and the complicated, but not unusual, family dynamic that often accompanies such a situation, see the archived articles on the Jehovah's Witnesses' website: Canadian Press (2002); Harrington (2002), and Williamson (2003).

2. Note here that I am critical of those who fail to engage patients about their spiritual or religious concerns and instead "turf" them to others. However, I applaud those providers who have these discussions with the patient and then partner with others, like Pastoral Care, as the need deepens. Collaboration is desirable; compartmentalization is not.

3. The Doctrine of Double Effect differentiates between actions and omissions that are intended and those that are merely foreseen. The morality of the action or omission rests on what is intended, not on those consequences that are merely foreseen. This principle is often used in just war theory, where the unintended (but foreseen) consequence of the deaths of noncombatants is justified by the acceptable intent of toppling an unjust regime, for example.

4. For an excellent discussion on the history of female circumcision in the United States, please see Webber (2005). For commentary on male circumcision, see Benatar and Benatar (2003).

WORKS CITED

Anderson, R. R. 2005. Case two: Religion and medicine.

Baggini, J., and M. Pym. 2005. End of life: The humanist view. *Lancet* 366: 1235–37.

Benatar, M., and D. Benatar. 2003. Between prophylaxis and child abuse: The ethics of neonatal male circumcision. *American Journal of Bioethics* 3 (2): 35–48.

Brown-Saltzman, K. A. 1994. Tending the spirit. *Oncology Nursing Forum* 21 (6): 1001–6.

Butler, S. M., H. G. Koenig, C. M. Puchalski, C. Cohen, and R. Sloan. 2003. *Is prayer good for your health? A critique of the scientific research.* Washington, DC: The Heritage Foundation.

Canadian Press. 2002. "Teen's transfusions must continue." http://www.watchtower informationservice.org/16ygirl2.htm (accessed October 28, 2003).

Chell, B. 1998. Competency: What it is, what it isn't, and why it matters. *Health care ethics: Critical issues for the 21st century*, ed. J. F. Monagle, and D. C. Thomasma. Gaithersburg, MD: Aspen.

Curlin, F. A., and D. E. Hall. 2005. Strangers or friends? A proposal for a new spirituality-in-medicine ethic. *Journal of General Internal Medicine* 20:370–74.

Curlin, F. A., C. J. Roach, R. Gorawara-Bhat, J. D. Lantos, and M. H. Chin. 2005. When patients choose faith over medicine. *Archives of Internal Medicine* 165:88–91.

Diekema, D. S., and the Committee on Bioethics. 2005. Responding to parental refusals of immunization of children. *Pediatrics* 115 (5): 1428–31.

Duckro, P. N., and P. R. Magaletta. 1994. The effect of prayer on physical health: Experimental evidence. *Journal of Religion and Health* 33 (3): 211–19.

Ehman, J. W., B. B. Ott, T. H. Short, R. C. Ciampa, and J. Hansen-Flaschen. 1999. Do patients want physicians to inquire about their spiritual or religious beliefs if they become gravely ill? *Archives of Internal Medicine* 159:1803–6.

Feudtner, C., J. Haney, and M. A. Dimmers. 2003. Spiritual care needs of hospitalized children and their families: A national survey of pastoral care providers' perceptions. *Pediatrics* 111 (1): e67–e72.

Furrow, B. R., T. L. Greaney, S. H. Johnson, T. S. Jost, and R. L. Schwartz. 2000. *Health law.* (accessed 2000).

Galanti, G. 1997. *Caring for patients from different cultures.* 2nd ed. Philadelphia: University of Pennsylvania Press.

Gordon, B. G. Jehovah's Witness refuses blood transfusion.

Groopman, J. 1997. *The measure of our days.* New York: Penguin Books.

———. 2004. *The anatomy of hope: How people prevail in the face of illness.* New York: Random House.

Handzo, G., and H. G. Koenig. 2004. Spiritual care: Whose job is it, anyway? *Southern Medical Journal* 97 (12): 1242–44.

Harrington, C. 2002. *Father shunned by family for defying faith to save child.* http://www.watchtowerinformationservice.org/fathershunned.htm (accessed October 28, 2003).

Hart, A., Jr., L. F. Tinker, D. J. Bowen, J. Satia-Abouta, and D. McLerran. 2004. Is religious orientation associated with fat and fruit/vegetable intake? *Journal of the American Dietetic Association* 104 (8): 1292–96.

Hester, D. M. 2001. *Community as healing.* Lanham, MD: Rowman & Littlefield.

Keown, D. 2005. End of life: The Buddhist view. *Lancet* 366:952–55.

Kliewer, S. 2004. Allowing spirituality into the healing process. *The Journal of Family Practice* 53 (8): 616–24.

LaPierre, L. L. 1994. The spirituality and religiosity of veterans. *Journal of Health Care Chaplaincy* 6 (1): 73–82.

Levin, J. 2003. Spiritual determinants of health and healing: An epidemiologic perspective on salutogenic mechanisms. *Alternative Therapies* 9 (6): 48–57.

Linnard-Palmer, L., and S. Kools. 2004. Parents' refusal of medical treatment based on religious and/or cultural beliefs: The law, ethical principles, and clinical implications. *Journal of Pediatric Nursing* 19 (5): 351–56.

Monroe, M. H., D. Bynum, B. Susi, N. Phifer, L. Schultz, M. Franco, C. D. MacLean, S. Cykert, and J. Garrett. 2003. Primary care physician preferences regarding spiritual behavior in medical practice. *Archives of Internal Medicine* 163:2751–56.

O'Neill, D. P., and E. K. Kenny. 1998. Spirituality and chronic illness. *Image: Journal of Nursing Scholarship* 30 (3): 275–79.

Palmer, R., D. Katerndahl, and J. Morgan-Kidd. 2004. A randomized trial of the effects of remote intercessory prayer: Interactions with personal beliefs on problem-specific outcomes and functional status. *The Journal of Alternative and Complementary Medicine* 10 (3): 438–48.

Pellegrino, E. 1979. Anatomy of a clinical encounter.

Puchalski, C. M. 2001. Reconnecting the science and art of medicine. *Academic Medicine* 76 (12): 1224–25.

Rubin, S. B. 1998. *When doctors say no: The battleground of medical futility.* Bloomington: Indiana University Press.

Trier, K. K., and A. Shupe. 1991. Prayer, religiosity, and healing in the heartland, USA: A research note. *Review of Religious Research* 32 (4): 351–58.

Vatuk, S. 2006. Dying in Hindu India. *Facing death: Where culture, religion, and medicine meet,* ed. H. M. Spiro, M. G. McCrea Curnen, and L. P. Wandel. New Haven, CT: Yale University Press.

Webber, S. 2005. *The "unnecessary" organ: A history of female circumcision and clitoridectomy in the United States, 1865–1995.* University of Nebraska Medical Center.

Williamson, K. 2003. "Bethany's battle rages a year after her death." http://www.watchtowerinformationservice.org/bethany.htm (accessed October 29, 2003).

ADDITIONAL RESOURCES

Committee on Doctrine of the National Conference of Catholic Bishops. 2001. *Ethical and religious directives for Catholic health care services.* http://www.usccb.org/bishops/directives.shtml (accessed December 29, 2005).

Dorff, E. N. 1998. *Matters of life and death: A Jewish approach to modern medical ethics.* Philadelphia: Jewish Publication Society.

Engelhardt, H. T., Jr., and A. S. Iltis. 2005. End-of-life: The traditional Christian view. *Lancet* 366:1045–49.

———. 2005. End-of-life: Jewish perspectives. *Lancet* 366:862–65.

Firth, S. 2005. End-of-life: A Hindu view. *Lancet* 366:682–86.

Joseph, J. C. 2002. *A chaplain's companion.* Judith C. Joseph.

Mackler, A. L., ed. 2000. *Life and death responsibilities in Jewish biomedical ethics.* New York: The Jewish Theological Seminary of America.

Markwell, H. 2005. End-of-life: A Catholic view. *Lancet* 366:1132–35.

McCormick, R. A. 1987. Health and medicine in the Catholic tradition. *Health/medicine and the faith traditions,* ed. M. E. Marty, and K. L. Vaux. New York: Crossroad.

Neuberger, J. 2004. *Caring for dying people of different faiths.* 3rd ed. Abingdon, UK: Radcliffe Medical Press.

Sachedina, A. 2005. End-of-life: The Islamic view. *Lancet* 366:774–79.

8

Ethics Consultation at the End of Life

Ideals, Rules, and Standards to Guide Decision Making

Lynn A. Jansen

KEY POINTS

1. Describe three common challenges that confront HECs called upon to respond to end-of-life ethical issues in the clinical setting.
2. Define two ideals that HECs might rely upon to supplement or strengthen the traditional assumptions about autonomy, privacy, and neutrality at the end of life.
3. Describe the difference between a rule and a standard, and define two rules and one standard commonly relied on by HECs to reason through difficult ethical problems at the end of life.
4. Describe how discontinuing medical interventions on the basis of biomedical futility differs from discontinuing medical interventions on the basis of a benefits/burdens assessment.

End-of-life decision making presents enduring problems in contemporary clinical ethics. While practices like physician assisted suicide and voluntary euthanasia continue to be hotly debated, bringing to the forefront the most controversial aspects of death and dying in the clinical setting, they are rarely the occasion for a hospital ethics consultation. In the clinical setting, ethical problems surrounding death and dying arise within a context in which there is general agreement about what is acceptable medical practice. HECs are typically called for consultation in order to help clinicians and family members select the most ethically appropriate option among the range of standard available medical interventions. This chapter identifies some pitfalls to be avoided in carrying out this task. It also discusses a number of important ethical rules and standards that should inform ethical decision making in the care of dying adults.

TRADITIONAL ASSUMPTIONS

Contemporary thinking about clinical ethics at the end of life is a response to relatively recent advances in medical technology. In the early 1970s, medical ethicists worried that technology was increasingly being used to prevent patients from dying "natural" deaths. This concern spawned a large literature that attempted to devise ethically defensible strategies for taming what was seen as the relentless technological imperative to control death (Beauchamp and Perlin 1978; Veatch 1976; Callahan 1993).

To understand contemporary end-of-life ethics, we need to begin by examining some of the key assumptions that informed these early efforts. I shall identify three of these assumptions here. As we shall see, an uncritical acceptance of these assumptions can distort ethical thinking at the end of life. The first assumption is what I shall call the *privacy of death*. It holds that patients should be free to "die on their own terms" and that death has a private meaning for each person. The second assumption is what I shall call the *centrality of autonomous agency*. It holds that patients who are dying have the capacity (and should be encouraged) to make use of legal instruments to ensure that their wishes are respected. The third assumption—I shall call it the *neutrality of clinical judgment* —holds that clinical judgment about the appropriate limits of medical interventions at the end of life should rest on general considerations of medical and technological efficacy, rather than on quality-of-life judgments made by the individual physician (Jansen 2006).[1]

These three assumptions, and the ideas underlying them, have defined a distinctive approach to end-of-life ethics that has been dominant for more than a quarter century. Those working in clinical ethics and serving on HECs are now sensitive to the moral value of encouraging patients to develop advance directives. They also understand the importance of incorporating the patient's values into end-of-life decision making and involving more perspectives than that of just the physician in the ethics consultation process. These are welcome and important developments. However, all too often, the ideas underlying the assumptions have been emphasized at the expense of other considerations relevant to sound end-of-life decision making.

It is crucial therefore to keep in mind that the assumptions remain merely a starting point. Without supplementation, they cannot aid HECs in addressing the full range of ethical issues that arise at the end of life in the modern hospital. This is true because the traditional assumptions often do not align with institutional realities of what it is like to die in the modern hospital. According to the Institute of Medicine, for example, more than 70 percent of those who die each year are elderly (Field and Cassell 1997). Many of these people will die hospitalized either because of, or while suffering from, advanced dementia. But patients at the end of life are also subject to various other pressures and disabilities. Many patients are depressed, psychologically isolated, fearful, and in pain. Others lack decisional capacity to various degrees and extents, and still others are financially burdened. All of these conditions can compromise the autonomous will of the dying patient.

Not surprisingly, these conditions also pose a challenge for HECs accustomed to relying on the centrality of autonomous agency. The centrality of autonomous agency enjoins members of HECs to address the difficult issues that surround end-of-life care by consulting the patient's desires, values, and wishes—in short, his or her will. And indeed, patients who are able to communicate their wishes, fears, and concerns about their own death should be encouraged and supported in doing so. But it is precisely when the will of the dying patient is compromised that HECs are most often called upon to guide clinicians, patients, and their families toward ethically responsible decisions. The fact that most dying patients do not have living wills or other advance directives makes this job all the more difficult. HECs who rely too heavily on the centrality of autonomous agency, then, will be ill equipped to help clinicians, patients, and their families make ethically sound decisions at the end of life.

Similar problems surround the traditional assumption about the privacy of death. Clinical ethicists are rightly trained to look to the family or "next of kin" to supply crucial information about the patient when the patient is no longer able to participate in decision making herself. Reliance on friends and relatives, even when one has not been specifically appointed to act as a healthcare proxy, is necessary to adopt the well-known perspectives of substituted judgment and best interest associated with surrogate decision making. Yet patients who die in the modern hospital frequently do not have stable support systems to play this role. Even when family members are present, there are often a number of factors, psychological and cultural, that make it difficult for them to participate in developing a plan of care for their loved one at the end of life. These factors pose yet another challenge for those accustomed to think of death as a private matter, one in which patients, in consultation with their family members, decide how to die with dignity.

One final challenge should be mentioned. Clinicians themselves often have difficulty coping with the death and dying of their patients. Despite the widespread recognition that patients need to take control of their own dying process, medical education still fails to "sufficiently prepare health professionals to recognize the final stages of illness, understand and manage their own emotional reaction to dying, construct effective strategies for care, and communicate sensitively to patients and those close to them" (Field and Cassell 1997). In effect, even when patients (or their families) are emotionally available and willing to participate in decision making at the end of life, clinicians often are not. Reliance on the neutrality of clinical judgment will do nothing to overcome this problem.

GUIDING IDEALS

To respond to these kinds of challenges, we need to supplement the traditional assumptions that have informed end-of-life ethics. If not supplemented, the traditional assumptions can mislead. But what supplementary ideals should inform the reasoning of HECs? Two ideals—*respect for persons* and *beneficence*—have been proposed as guides. These ideals capture the truth in the traditional assumptions, but in addition, they can be relied on to address a range of ethical problems clinicians who care for dying patients are likely to encounter in the modern hospital.

The ideal of respect for persons is frequently associated with the imperative to honor patient autonomy. Patients at the end of life, like other patients, have desires about what kinds of medical interventions they would like to receive. The importance of respecting these desires underlies a number of negative and positive duties.[2] When patients are able to communicate their wishes and desires to their clinicians, then these wishes normally should be respected. And when patients have decision-making capacity, clinicians often have no difficulty ascertaining the relevant negative and positive duties they have toward their patients. But while respecting patient autonomy is obviously a crucial part of what it means to respect a person, it does not exhaust the content of the ideal (Velleman 2006). It is widely recognized that clinicians should not simply defer to the autonomous desires of their patients, whatever these desires may be. A surgeon who acts on a patient's request to amputate a limb is unnecessarily acting wrongly, even if the patient has decisional capacity. And, as noted above, many patients who die in the modern hospital are in no position to express their autonomous wishes with respect to their medical treatments.

These simple examples show that the ideal of respect for persons requires more than honoring patient autonomy. It also requires valuing persons as individuals with dignity. This expression refers to the status of human beings as deserving respect and that the respect owed to them is independent of any particular status they occupy or physical capabilities they happen to have (Velleman 2006). In Kantian moral theory, this respect is grounded in the fact that human beings have a rational nature (Kant 1964). The duty to show respect for this rational nature bars us from doing certain things to others, as well as to ourselves.

The second guiding ideal is that of beneficence. This ideal directs clinicians to promote the well-being of their patients. To do this, they must promote the interests of their patients. But what are the relevant interests? It is helpful to divide patient interests into two broad categories: those that concern the experiences of the patient (phenomenological interests) and those that do not (nonphenomenological interests).[3] Alleviation of fear, pain, and other types of physical symptoms are often the most pressing phenomenological interests patients have when facing death. However, terminally ill patients have nonphenomenological interests as well.

Nonphenomenological interests are not well characterized in terms of maintaining a patient's comfort. For this reason, they can conflict (or appear to conflict) with the phenomenological interests a patient may have. For example, a terminally ill patient may believe that it is more important to remain alert than have his pain fully controlled.

Or, perhaps a patient believes that his religious convictions require that he not forego burdensome medical interventions that may prolong his life, but offer no hope for recovery.

Like the ideal of respect for persons, the requirements of the ideal of beneficence can be a source of ethical conflict. The interests of patients can remain unmet because their clinician believes that a full response to these interests would conflict with the ideal of respect for persons discussed above or with other moral commitments that the clinician may have. We will discuss this kind of conflict in greater detail below.

MEDIATING STANDARDS AND RULES

The two ideals we have been discussing, respect for persons and beneficence, can help to orient thinking about the nature of the ethical issue one confronts in the clinical setting. But these ideals are abstract. To apply them in the hospital, HECs must have recourse to mediating rules or standards. These rules and standards intercede between the theoretical ideals discussed above and the concrete problems to which HECs are asked to respond.

There are a number of different rules and standards that HECs might rely on to work through difficult ethical dilemmas at the end of life. Obviously, they cannot all be discussed here. Instead, I will focus on three of the most important, clarifying their meaning and showing how they can be properly applied to actual cases. These are:

1. The standard of deliberation
2. The rule of double effect
3. The rule of medical futility

This standard and these rules are controversial and often misunderstood in the clinical context. However, when carefully formulated, they can provide guidance in resolving ethical issues that are likely to arise at the end of life, given the institutional realities we have discussed.

There is not a sharp distinction between a rule and a standard. As I will use these terms here, a rule articulates permissions and requirements. A rule with respect to truth-telling, for example, identifies when one is permitted to lie and when one is required to tell the truth. In contrast, a standard articulates an end or aspiration to which one should aim to achieve. A standard of artistic excellence, for example, identifies a target to aim at, even if it does not set out the precise steps for hitting the target in terms of permissions and requirements. Sometimes the application of a rule may be unclear, doing little more than gesturing toward considerations that need to be taken into account. Sometimes the pursuit of a standard will require one to take very specific steps. That is why the distinction between them is not sharp.

A. The Standard of Deliberation

The standard of deliberation relates to shared decision making in medicine. Shared decision making in medicine is a collaborative process between the clinician and the patient (Emanuel and Emanuel 1992; Brock 1993). As is now widely recognized, shared decision making is important in most aspects of the medical encounter. However, it is critically important for decision making at the end of life (Emanuel 1995). In this context, ethically sound decisions about what course of action to pursue depend heavily on how well the clinical team is able to reach an understanding of the patient's values and coax them into clarity. Indeed, studies show that the quality of care that patients receive at the end of life correlates strongly with the willingness of clinicians to engage in discussions with their patients about prognosis, goals of care, advance directives, when to forego medical interventions, and concerns about family support (SUPPORT Study 1995).

The idea of shared decision making, however, does not prescribe a specific formula for interaction between clinicians and patients. The proper stance for the clinician to take will depend on many variables, such as the temperament and educational background of the patient. Nonetheless, the extent to which shared decision making serves the ideals of respect for persons and beneficence will depend, in large measure, on the type and quality of deliberation that takes place between the clinical team and patients and families. The standard of deliberation provides guidance on this matter.

The standard can be formulated as follows:

> Clinicians should take an active role in enabling patients and families to make medical decisions in a reasoned, well-informed manner that accurately reflects the concerns and values of the patient.

The standard of deliberation does not prescribe specific requirements. It is a standard, not a rule. But it does point toward a kind of
excellence in the clinical encounter.

According to this standard, the role of the clinician in shared decision making is not merely to inform the patient of the range of medical options. Rather, it asks clinicians to take a more active role in
stimulating patients and families to think about how the patient's
values bear on medical decisions in a reasoned and well-informed
manner (Jansen 2006; Berdes and Emanuel 2006).

The standard of deliberation thus contrasts with the assumption of
clinical neutrality. Clinicians who care for dying patients are often
tempted to interpret their role as simply an information provider.
They are to inform patients (or families) of the range of available
clinical options and then wait for the patients (or families) to decide
for themselves which course should be undertaken. The provision of
relevant information is obviously important, but if a clinician merely
provides information, he or she will fail to provide the ethical guidance that patients and families need in making crucial decisions at
the end of life.

To appreciate these points more fully, consider the following case.

Case 1

Mrs. A. is a forty-nine-year-old woman with terminal breast cancer that has metastasized to the brain. Over the past four months, Mrs. A's decision-making capacity
has gradually waned, until finally she is no longer able to make decisions for herself. Recently, Mrs. A. has also stopped taking adequate hydration and nutrition. She
left no living will, and she assigned no healthcare proxy. Her sister (Beth) has been
acting as her surrogate decision maker. Beth is confused and distraught over what
she views as a "sudden change" in her sister's condition. Beth believes that her sister should be fed, but she does not want to cause her unnecessary suffering. The attending physician tells Beth that her sister could have tube feedings as a supplement. However, the consulting surgeon disagrees. He tells Beth that the fact that her
sister has stopped eating is a natural part of the dying process. He also tells Beth
that he would not want a tube feeding for himself in this situation. The attending
physician is irate. He believes that the decision to use tube feedings in the case of
Mrs. A. is "Beth's call." An ethics consultation is called.

Case 1 illustrates several general problems that confront end-of-life decision making between physicians, patients, and family members.
First, end-of-life decision making involves patients and their families
in a range of new experiences. Denial or fear may make it difficult or

impossible for patients and their family members in these circumstances to process the information that is made available to them. In Case 1, for example, Beth's anxiety could prevent her from reasoning in a way appropriate to the role of a surrogate decision maker. Second, patients at the end of life often do not have clearly formed values, and mistakes can be made in translating their wishes into particular treatment decisions. In Case 1, Mrs. A. left no advance directive.

Third, terminally ill patients frequently lack full decision-making capacity. This brings surrogates and healthcare proxies into the decision-making process. Proper respect for the patient requires the surrogate decision maker to reason from a distinctive perspective— that of *substituted judgment*, or when this is not available, that of *best interests*. Understanding and adopting these perspectives frequently requires support from physicians and the clinical team. In Case 1, an ethics consultation was called because the physicians had provided no guidance to Beth on this matter. The surgeon, adopting a stance of clinical neutrality, simply informed Beth that she was the one responsible for making the decision about the tube feeding. A more deliberative response would have required the surgeon to initiate a dialogue with Beth to determine whether Mrs. A had ever expressed views about dying in general and tube feedings in particular. This might require him to explain to her the perspective of substituted judgment and its importance to surrogate decision making. If this dialogue determined that Mrs. A had never expressed her values on this matter, then the physician should direct Beth to consider whether a tube feeding would in fact best advance Mrs. A's medical and nonmedical interests at this time.[4]

As Case 1 illustrates, many ethics consults are called simply because clinicians fail to deliberate with family members about how to apply the perspectives of substituted judgment and best interests and how these perspectives relate to appropriate medical treatment. Studies show that clinicians have a difficult time engaging in shared decision making at the end of life (Field and Cassell 1997). One reason for this may have to do with the lack of exposure clinicians receive in their medical training to death and dying. However, an additional compounding reason may be that clinicians fail to understand how the standard of deliberation can be used to help patients and families set reasonable and achievable goals at the end of life.

HECs have an important role to play in helping clinicians and their patients realize the standard of deliberation. HECs need to be aware of the reasons why shared decision making can fail at the end of life. They also need to be skilled in helping clinicians move from simply providing information to a more deliberative approach. The standard of deliberation directs clinicians, patients, and family members to initiate a dialogue about how the patient's values and preferences bear on the available interventions. The point of such a dialogue should be to help clinicians, patients, and families come to reasoned decisions about the treatment options that are available and the treatment that should be pursued. It also provides a structured opportunity for all involved to identify and correct mistaken beliefs about interventions and their role in staving off the dying process. For example, family members of dying patients sometimes mistakenly believe that cardiopulmonary resuscitation will permanently forestall death. Deliberative discussion with the family and clinical team can help identify and correct such mistaken beliefs.

The standard of deliberation serves the two ideals mentioned in the previous section. It respects persons by enabling the clinical team or surrogate decision maker to further the autonomous wishes of dying patients. It promotes beneficence by helping to ensure that dying patients are not subjected to unnecessary and unwanted medical interventions. Indeed, given the complexity of the issues that patients, clinicians, and families face as patients approach death, a strong case exists for holding that the standard of deliberation is the fundamental ethical standard for guiding ethics consultation at the end of life.

B. The Rule of Double Effect

While fundamental, the standard of deliberation only goes so far. Specifically, the standard of deliberation does not directly address the limits of a clinician's obligation to comply with the wishes of patients or family members that emerge from shared decision making. These limits are important, since many of the ethical concerns that arise at the end of life have to do with them. Ethically responsible decision making, therefore, also depends on the application of relevant ethical rules.

One rule that is particularly important at the end of life is the rule of double effect. This rule, as we shall see, is vital for the proper treatment of the pain and suffering of terminally ill patients. According to the rule of double effect[5]:

> An action, such as a medical intervention, with two foreseeable effects, one good and one bad, is morally permitted if (1) the action is undertaken with the intention of achieving only the good effect, and (2) the action is undertaken for a proportionate reason.

The rule of double effect is important, but it is easily misunderstood, and clinicians often are uncertain how to apply it.

As the above formulation makes clear, the rule of double effect has two components. The first component rests on the distinction between an intended and a merely foreseen effect of an intervention. The nature and moral significance of this distinction has given rise to much controversy in medical ethics (Quill et al. 1997a). Still, understanding the distinction between intended and foreseen effects is crucial for the proper treatment of terminally ill patients. The second component expresses the requirement of proportionality. This component is widely accepted. Even critics of the first component of the rule of double effect accept the idea that medical interventions with a bad effect should be undertaken only for a proportionate reason (Quill et al. 1997b; Jansen and Sulmasy 2002).

Both components can be clarified by considering the vexed issue of how clinicians should respond to the pain and suffering of terminally ill patients. The laws of most countries forbid clinicians from intentionally killing their patients. And, even if doing so is legally permitted, many clinicians believe that it is wrong for them intentionally to kill, or assist in the death, of their patients. These realities have contributed to the widely documented fact of the undertreatment of pain at the end of life. As the case below illustrates, many clinicians are reluctant to prescribe appropriate doses of medication to control the pain and suffering of their patients either because they fear legal reprisal or because they believe that doing so would implicate them in the death of their patients (Quill and Meier 2006; Lo and Rubenfeld 2005).

Case 2

Mr. B. is a thirty-year-old man with end-stage osteogenic sarcoma. Cure is no longer possible after years of struggle with surgery, radiation, and chemotherapy. In expert hands, he has required increasing doses of morphine for pain relief. However, he has now developed very bothersome myoclonus as a side effect of protracted high-dose opioids. He is now bed-bound, dyspneic, and near death. Standard doses of muscle relaxants and benzodiazepines have not controlled the myoclonus, and despite adjuvant pain treatments, his pain is increasing and responds only to increasing opioids, thereby increasing his myoclonus. He is groggy, but alert. The physician is aware that increasing doses of benzodiazepines can control the myoclonus, but he is also aware that the doses required to achieve this end would also precipitate a coma and even death. Since the physician has principled objections to physician-assisted suicide and euthanasia, he calls an ethics consult to discuss whether palliative sedation in this case would be ethically justified.[6]

When administering pain medication to terminally ill patients in cases like Case 2, clinicians often worry about becoming implicated in the patient's death.

How might the two components of the rule of double effect help clinicians think more clearly about such matters? According to the first component of the rule, administering high, and even lethal, doses of pain medication can be done with the intention to control the patient's pain—an admittedly "good" effect. The death of the patient—a typically "bad" effect in these cases—can be understood to be a foreseen, but unintended, effect of the medical intervention.

Critics of the rule of double effect sometimes question the sharpness of the distinction between foreseen and intended effects. Clinicians, after all, may intend both to control the patient's pain and to hasten his death (Lo and Rubenfeld 2005). In other cases, clinicians may be unclear about what exactly is the intended effect of their intervention. A full response to these worries is not possible here. But a few remarks are in order. To begin with, a large number of clinicians believe that while it is ethically appropriate to administer pain medication, it is not ethically appropriate to intentionally hasten the death of their patients. This is the situation for the physician in Case 2. For these clinicians, the distinction between an intended and a merely foreseen effect of a medical intervention is vitally important. The fact that some clinicians may not object to intentionally killing their patients does not detract from this point.[7] Secondly, in situations where clinicians are unclear about what their intentions are, it is plausible to hold that they have a duty to clarify them. As we have seen, clinicians sometimes have difficulty confronting the reality that their patients die, and medical training often fails to prepare them adequately to manage the symptoms of their dying patients. Frustration and feelings of professional inadequacy in helping the patient die well can further blur clinical intentions. All of these factors likely contribute to the ambiguity of clinical intentions with respect to the rule of double effect. Accordingly, HECs have a role to play in helping clinicians to distinguish the intended from merely foreseen effects of medical interventions at the end of life.

Good intentions, of course, are not sufficient for good medical practice. Medical interventions also need to be proportionately undertaken. This means that the medical intervention must be appropriate given the patient's condition and that the good to be achieved by the intervention must be of sufficient weight to justify the imposition of the foreseen bad effect. This brings us to the second component of the rule of double effect. While less controversial, this component is also subject to misunderstanding, particularly when it is applied to decision making at the end of life. In responding to the pain and suffering of the terminally ill, what exactly does it mean to speak of a proportionate reason for an intervention?

It is widely acknowledged that the need to alleviate the pain and suffering of terminally ill patients is a reason of sufficient weight to justify high-risk interventions (Hallenbeck 2000; Quill and Byock 2000; Quill and Brody 1996). In general, the more intense the patient's pain and suffering, the easier it is to justify high-risk interventions to control it. But proportionality, in this context, does not refer simply to the intensity of the pain and suffering of a patient. It must also refer to its underlying cause. Here we confront a pitfall that clinicians need to be careful to avoid. When it comes to treating patients at the end of life, clinicians may be tempted to sum up the different kinds of suffering a particular patient is experiencing and treat it all in the same way (Quill et al. 1997a). This runs afoul of the proportionality component of the rule of double effect (Jansen and Sulmasy 2002; Lo and Rubenfeld 2005). To see this, consider the distinction between physical pain and existential suffering. High doses of narcotics can be an appropriate response to unmanaged physical pain, such as the myoclonus experienced by the patient in Case 2, but it is not an appropriate response to existential suffering. A terminally ill patient who suffers from depression or despair, for example, will not benefit from being placed into a barbiturate coma. With respect to patients who are not terminally ill, this point is perfectly obvious. Physicians readily distinguish the despair that accompanies the loss of a limb from the physical pain associated with that loss. And no competent physician would treat the former with medications appropriate for the latter. But at the end of life, clinicians can lose sight of this basic point. They may be inclined to view terminally ill patients as patients who have no interests in restoration at all (Jansen and Sulmasy 2002). While it is true that the terminally ill cannot be restored to physical health, it does not follow that their nonphenomenological interests (psychological, experiential, and spiritual) cannot be restored. Failure to attend to these interests appropriately fails to show proper respect for persons.

The proportionality component of the rule of double effect can help clinicians avoid this pitfall. When properly understood and applied, it directs clinicians first to discriminate between different kinds of pain and suffering and then to prescribe treatments that are proportionate to the kinds of pain and suffering present. The terminally ill, while they do not have much time left to live, remain persons who are entitled to the respect that is due all rational agents. The rule of double effect thus not only helps clinicians honor the ideal of beneficence, but also the ideal of respect for persons.

The rule of double effect cannot resolve all the ethical dilemmas that arise at the end of life. But it can provide guidance in thinking through a range of cases concerning the treatment of the pain and suffering of terminally ill patients. These cases frequently require clinicians to undertake interventions that have both good and bad effects, and sometimes they require clinicians to decide whether a high-risk intervention, such as administering a potentially lethal dose of pain medication, is an appropriate and proportionate response to the pain and suffering of their patients.

C. The Rule of Medical Futility

Unlike the rule of double effect, there is currently no established consensus in the medical community on how to define medical futility. Nonetheless, clinicians and family members caring for terminally ill patients do sometimes find themselves attempting to justify limiting or discontinuing medical treatment based on what we might call the *rule of medical futility*. According to the rule of medical futility:

A medical intervention should not be undertaken if it will be ineffective in achieving its proposed biomedical end or will cause the patient to experience continual or repeated need for the intervention over a very short period of time before death.

At the end of life, the rule of medical futility comes into play in a number of circumstances. Sometimes a terminally ill patient does not have decision-making capacity, lacks an advance directive, and does not have a surrogate decision maker. In this kind of case, a clinician might wonder when it is appropriate for him to discontinue medical treatment. In other situations, a terminally ill patient or the surrogate decision maker for such a patient requests that an intervention be undertaken or continued that the clinician believes is no longer medically appropriate. In these contexts, clinicians often appeal to the rule of medical futility to justify their decisions. But, of course, not all decisions to discontinue treatment can be justified according to this rule. The difficulty, then, is to figure out how to characterize what makes a medical intervention futile.

Families and clinicians often disagree over what it means to describe an intervention as medically futile (Schneiderman et al. 1990). These disagreements can be especially difficult to deal with when they occur at the end of a patient's life. Without an operational definition of futility to guide decision making in the clinical context, futility judgments run the risk of appearing arbitrary and unmotivated.

Hospital administrators and ethics committees sometimes draft institutional policies on medical futility as a practical remedy to this problem.[8] Futility policies serve an important legitimizing role in the clinical context because they require those involved in the care of patients to base their futility judgments on uniform, publicly defended standards rather than their own idiosyncratic ideas of the concept. While the mere existence of a futility policy will not do away with all futility conflicts, it can provide a framework for keeping all parties focused on the issues at hand. When carefully drafted, a futility policy can help clinicians and families honor the two ideals—respect for persons and beneficence—that we have been discussing.

While there is disagreement on the matter,[9] a strong case can be made that futility policies should articulate a clear and relatively narrow definition of medical futility. Consider the following definition (which is implied by the above formulation of the rule of medical futility):

> Medical futility refers to the clinical judgment that, to a reasonable degree of medical certitude, based on the patient's current clinical circumstances, the proposed intervention(s) will not achieve its specific biomedical goal or will cause the patient to experience continual or repeated need for the intervention over a very short period of time before death.[10]

This definition directs physicians and families to evaluate a proposed medical intervention in terms of its effectiveness in achieving its specific biomedical goal. It directs attention away from extrinsic considerations, such as how much the intervention would cost.

The definition also directs physicians to think of futility in terms of specific interventions, rather than in terms of the patient's overall medical condition. For example, applying the above definition, a physician might correctly describe cardiopulmonary resuscitation for a particular patient as futile. However, it would not be correct for her to describe the patient's *condition* as futile. This distinction is important, but frequently overlooked. When properly observed, the distinction allows the clinical team to stop providing some particular treatment regarded as futile while still recognizing that the patient can appropriately continue to receive other medical care. A judgment of medical futility, properly understood, does not relieve the clinical team of its positive duties to promote the patient's well-being, such as to provide palliative care.

> **Case 3**
>
> Mr. C. is a seventy-four-year-old man with anoxic brain damage following a cardiac arrest in his home. He has been comatose since his admission to the hospital six months ago. His condition is slowly deteriorating. He is presently experiencing renal failure and is on dialysis. He is also ventilator-dependent. Mr. C. left no living will. He has no family or surrogate decision maker. The clinical team has started to discuss the possibility of limiting certain medical interventions. May they discontinue the ventilator or the dialysis? Is it permissible for them to write a DNR order, thus withholding cardiopulmonary resuscitation if the patient's heart stops again? An ethics consultation is called.

According to the rule of medical futility that we have provided, it is not permissible on grounds of medical futility to discontinue the ventilator or dialysis in Case 3. The reason for this judgment is that both of these interventions (at least in this case) effectively achieve their biomedical purpose.[11] This is not the case with the DNR order, however. According to studies reported by American Medical Association's Council on Ethical and Judicial Affairs (CEJA), the "outcome of CPR is dependent upon the nature and severity of the patient's underlying illness prior to cardiopulmonary arrest" (CEJA 1991). It is for this reason that the American Medical Association has recommended that resuscitation not be attempted if the treating physician judges that the procedure would be futile (CEJA 1991).[12] In Case 3, given the gravity of the patient's condition coupled with his previous heart failure, it is not unreasonable to conclude that CPR would not achieve its biomedical goal. The decision to withhold cardiopulmonary resuscitation to Mr. C., therefore, could reasonably be justified on grounds of medical futility.[13]

As stated above, a hospital policy on medical futility should define medical futility in clear and relatively narrow terms. The judgment that a particular medical intervention is futile is a clinical judgment, one that clinicians, not healthcare proxies or family members, typically have expertise to make. While judgments of futility ultimately rest on a physician's assessment that a particular medical intervention will not achieve its biomedical goal, HECs should avoid drafting (or endorsing) policies that permit physicians to execute futility determinations without informing family members. In Case 3, there were no family members present. But when family members are present, there are both moral and prudential reasons for physicians to inform them that a judgment of medical futility has been reached. Respect for family members who care for a dying patient requires the physician to keep them informed of all major medical decisions. In addition, there is potential for unnecessary conflict between the clinical team and the family if clinicians make futility judgments without informing all interested parties. Clinicians and family members should be encouraged to discuss these issues early on so that all parties are aware that the medical team is not obligated to pursue futile medical interventions.

The rule of medical futility provides one important justification for withholding or withdrawing medical interventions. Once the definition of futility has been made reasonably precise, the application of the rule to particular cases can be based on general considerations of medical and technological efficacy, thus avoiding quality-of-life evaluations. In this way, the rule of medical futility sits well with the neutrality of clinical judgment discussed in section A.

Matters become more controversial, however, if the judgment to withhold or withdraw a medical intervention is not based on the rule of medical futility. In Case 3, as we have seen, the withdrawal of the ventilator cannot be justified on grounds of medical futility, but it might be justified nonetheless on other grounds. It might be justified, for example, on grounds that the burdens of the intervention outweigh its benefits. It is crucial not to conflate benefits/burdens assessments with assessments of medical futility. Benefits/burdens assessments rest on quality-of-life judgments that clinicians have no special expertise to make. When the judgment to discontinue an intervention is based on a benefits/burdens assessment, it is appropriate for clinicians to consult, deliberate with, and often defer to, the judgments of healthcare proxies or family members with respect to the wishes and best interests of the patient. The same is not true of judgments of medical futility, providing medical futility is defined in clear and relatively narrow terms.

SOME FURTHER COMPLEXITIES: WITHHOLDING AND WITHDRAWING MEDICAL INTERVENTIONS

Benefits/burdens assessments can provide another justification for withholding or withdrawing life-sustaining medical interventions. Nevertheless, clinicians may worry that withdrawing an intervention that was *not* futile would constitute an ethically impermissible act of killing. Is this worry well founded?

A. Killing and Letting Die

The withdrawal of a life-sustaining intervention can be done without the intention to kill the patient. The rule of double effect, as we have seen, shows how it is possible knowingly to cause a death without intending it. But the rule of double effect is silent on whether a moral distinction can be made between killing, on the one hand, and letting die, on the other. In the context of end-of-life medical care, it might be thought that there is, in fact, a significant moral difference between killing a patient and merely letting her die. Further, it might be thought that acts of withdrawing a nonfutile medical intervention fall on one side of this line and acts of withholding a non-futile medical intervention fall on the other.

These points raise complex issues. Let us begin by assuming that, other things being equal, an act of withdrawing a medical intervention and an act of withholding a medical intervention are morally equivalent (CEJA 1998–1999; Beauchamp and Childress 1994). Then we will discuss whether this assumption is defensible.

Nonfutile medical interventions can be withheld or withdrawn for a variety of reasons. First, a competent patient has the right to refuse unwanted medical treatment, even if the treatment would be effective. Second, a patient's surrogate decision maker can reject medical interventions that he or she judges would either be contrary to the patient's wishes and values or not be in the patient's best interests. This latter judgment will require a general overall assessment of the impact a proposed intervention would have on the quality of life of the patient. Third, under some circumstances, a physician can reject medical interventions if he judges that they would impose an unfavorable balance of benefits and burdens on the patient. These circumstances chiefly include cases in which the patient lacks decisional capacity and there is no legally appointed healthcare proxy or family member. This is was the situation in Case 3 discussed above. Here the physician can permissibly discontinue the dialysis or ventilator of Mr. C., provided that such interventions are disproportionately burdensome and therefore contrary to the patient's best interest. The justification for the discontinuation of these interventions would not appeal to the rule of medical futility, but rather to the ideal of beneficence that should inform medical practice.

Still, as Case 3 illustrates, physicians may be more reluctant to withdraw a medical intervention than to withhold one. Refusing to provide cardiopulmonary resuscitation would simply allow Mr. C. to die, while discontinuing the ventilator, it may be thought, would kill him. But is this thought correct? Is it right to characterize the withdrawal of the ventilator as an instance of killing? Instances of withdrawing aid, such as the removal of the ventilator in Case 3, are plausibly characterized as an allowing to die, rather than an act of killing. To see this, we can distinguish the potential causes of death from the defensive efforts undertaken to combat those causes. If these defensive efforts are judged to be ineffective or excessively burdensome, then they can be withdrawn. Their withdrawal will, in turn, let the patient die from the original underlying causes of death. This will be true, even though it is correct to describe the withdrawal of the aid as an active intervention.

Of course, it matters who withdraws the intervention. For the withdrawal of aid to constitute a letting die, rather than a killing, it must be the case that the agent who withdraws the aid is the same agent who provided it. For example, if some third party were to discontinue the ventilator in Case 3, then this would plausibly constitute an act of killing. In the context of the hospital, however, the agent providing the aid can be considered to include all the members of the medical team who are entitled to provide and withdraw aid (Kamm 1996).

This analysis suggests that both withdrawals and withholdings of medical interventions can qualify as cases of letting die. Coming to see that this is the case can help clinicians and family members overcome anxieties about actively discontinuing medical treatment. If the burdens of a particular medical intervention outweigh its benefits, then the decision to withdraw it is a decision to let the patient die, rather than a decision to kill him.[14]

B. Responding to Conflicts

We have been focusing on cases in which either there is no surrogate decision maker present or there is agreement between the clinical team and the surrogate decision maker. Unfortunately, clinicians and surrogates do not always agree, even after sincere deliberation and even after an ethics consultation has been called. When disagreement cannot be resolved, we might wonder whether physicians are always required to defer to the surrogate decision maker's judgment of the benefits/burdens assessment.

When the physician and the surrogate disagree about whether a proposed intervention would be, on balance, beneficial to the patient, then in general, the physician should respect the wishes of the surrogate. Almost any judgment that a medical intervention is disproportionately burdensome is considerably more controversial than a judgment of medical futility. There is wide scope for reasonable disagreement on these matters. However, if the surrogate insists that an intervention be undertaken that no reasonable physician[15] would judge to be in the patient's best interests, then the physician is not required to provide the intervention (CEJA 1998–1999). The difficulty, of course, is determining when a surrogate's request is beyond the pale.

The difficult case occurs when the requested intervention would not be medically futile, but the physician believes that no reasonable case can be made that its potential benefits would outweigh its potential burdens to the patient. Famously, such a situation was present in the case of Helga Wanglie (Beauchamp and Childress 1994). Wanglie suffered severe anoxic encephalopathy and was in a persistent vegetative state. Her physician and her surrogate decision maker could not agree on whether the patient's ventilator should be turned off. Strictly speaking, the ventilator was achieving its specific biomedical purpose and therefore it was not futile. Nevertheless, the physician believed that it was inappropriate to continue with the medical intervention. The ethics committee at his hospital agreed.

In cases like Wanglie's, the physician may be morally justified in challenging the surrogate's request to provide the intervention. The basis of such a challenge must be that the physician's duty of beneficence to the patient takes precedence over his duty to respect the surrogate's decision-making authority. The physician in this case held that the respirator was not beneficial treatment "in that it could not heal [Wanglie's] lungs, palliate her suffering, or enable [her] to experience the benefit of the life afforded by respirator support" (Beauchamp and Childress 1994). And, obviously, if a treatment has no prospect for benefit, then it cannot have a favorable benefits/burdens ratio. Still, cases like Wanglie's illustrate the exception, not the rule. For, as noted above, physicians do not have special expertise in making quality-of-life judgments with respect to their patients. Assuming that the surrogate is acting in good faith, physicians should, accordingly, be very reluctant to challenge the surrogate's assessment of the benefits and burdens of a proposed intervention.

Conflicts between physicians and surrogate decision makers should, if at all possible, be resolved within the hospital. An ethics consultation should aim to resolve these conflicts. However, if disagreement is intractable, physicians face a difficult situation. They might consider transferring the patient to another institution that expresses a willingness to provide the medical intervention. There is no guarantee, of course, that there will be such an institution. Alternatively, a physician can challenge the surrogate's decision-making authority in court. This option should be done as a last resort and with great reluctance. Courts generally do not like to intervene in such matters, and the process of going to court may impose considerable hardship on the physician and the patient's family.

CONCLUSION

End-of-life decision making is rarely easy for anyone involved. The difficulties become even more pronounced when the dying patient lacks decision-making capacity and has no family members or surrogate decision makers to speak on his or her behalf. In these situations, traditional assumptions about end-of-life decision making, which include the centrality of autonomy, the privacy of death, and the neutrality of clinical judgment, ring hollow, leaving clinicians ill-equipped to help their patients die well.

This chapter has focused on a range of ethical ideals, rules, and standards designed to supplement the traditional assumptions. It has not purported to offer an exhaustive treatment of all the issues surrounding the ethics of death and dying. The chapter also has not discussed the legal considerations that bear on these issues and that vary from jurisdiction to jurisdiction. More modestly, the goal of the chapter has been to introduce and critically discuss some important and difficult topics that HECs come into contact with on a daily basis in the clinical setting.[16]

FOR FURTHER REFLECTION

1. Despite its importance, clinicians often have difficulty engaging their patients and patients' families in shared decision making at the end of life. Describe three obstacles to shared decision making. How might your HEC assist clinicians, patients, and families in overcoming these obstacles?
2. This chapter discusses some of the ethical issues associated with an uncritical acceptance of clinical neutrality. Discuss how the assumption of clinical neutrality manifests itself in your own clinical setting. Consider, also, whether there is a difference between tolerance and neutrality in the clinical setting. If so, how might HECs help clinicians appreciate this difference in their approach to patients and families at the end of life?
3. Discuss the rule of double effect. Does this rule have practical application for end-of-life care?

NOTES

1. The ideas presented in this section were previously developed in my introduction to *Death in the Clinic* (Jansen 2006).

2. Positive duties require some kind of action. The duty to provide CPR to a patient in cardiac arrest is a positive duty. In contrast, negative duties forbid actions. The duty to refrain from imposing unwanted medical treatment on a patient is a negative duty.

3. The discussion of phenomenological and nonphenomenological interests is developed from L. A. Jansen, B. Johnston, and D. P. Sulmasy, "Ethical Issues," in *A Clinical Guide to Supportive and Palliative Care for HIV/AIDS* (2003).

4. State laws differ with regard to the "burden of proof" required for discontinuing tube feedings. New York State, for example, requires "clear and convincing evidence" that the patient would not have wanted to receive tube feedings before the feeding may be legally withdrawn. Ethics consultants should be aware of the relevant laws in their own state.

5. In the medical ethics literature, the rule of double effect often takes on a more complex formulation. For example, T. L. Beauchamp and J. F. Childress (1994, 207) define the rule as the following four components: (1) the nature of the act, (2) the agent's intention, (3) the distinction between means and effects, and (4) proportionality between the good effect and the bad effect. The two components I focus on in this chapter are the ones that are most relevant to end-of-life ethics, and nothing is lost from an ethical point of view from my way from framing the rule.

6. This case is taken from L. A. Jansen, B. Johnston, and D. P. Sulmasy, "Ethical Issues," in *A Clinical Guide to Supportive and Palliative Care for HIV/AIDS* (2003).

7. The point here is not that HECs should try to make clinicians feel better about their decisions, irrespective of the merits of these decisions. Rather, the point is that HECs may need to take seriously the actual moral views of clinicians in order to advise them to make decisions that are in the best interests of patients. Persuading a clinician that the distinction between intending the death and merely foreseeably bringing about the death of a patient is not as morally important as he thinks may not be a realistic option in the circumstances of the clinical setting.

8. The Council on Ethical and Judicial Affairs recommends that all hospitals adopt a policy on medical futility. See AMA policy E-2.037 "Medical Futility in End-of-life Care," http://www.ama-assn.org/ama/pub/category/8390.html (accessed November 1, 2005).

9. See, for example, the discussion of a proceduralist/consensus-driven notion of futility in T. Tomlinson and D. Czlonka, "Futility and Hospital Policy" (2000, 419–429).

10. This is the definition of futility used in the futility policy relied upon by St. Vincent's Medical Center, Manhattan. The policy was drafted by the members of the hospital ethics committee and affirmed as hospital policy in 1998.

11. It is possible, as we will see below, that the clinical team is justified in discontinuing these interventions. If so, the justification for doing so will rest on a benefits/burdens assessment and not on grounds of medical futility.

12. See, for example, CEJA: "Guidelines for the Appropriate Use of Do-Not-Resuscitate Orders" (1991).

13. This is not to say that dialysis or mechanical ventilation could *never* satisfy the rule of futility. It is only in this particular case that they do not satisfy the rule.

14. Much has been written on the withdrawing/withholding aid distinction. I have followed Kamm's discussion. For a different view see S. Kagan, *The Limits of Morality* (1989, 116–21).

15. The reasonable physician standard is meant to underscore that the judgment should be a shared professional judgment and not a physician's own personal judgment.

16. Thanks to D. Micah Hester for very helpful comments and criticisms on successive drafts of this chapter.

WORKS CITED

Beauchamp, T. L., and J. Childress. 1994. *Principles of biomedical ethics*. 4th ed. New York: Oxford University Press.

Beauchamp, T. L., and S. Perlin. 1978. *Ethical issues in death and dying*. Englewood Cliffs, NJ: Prentice-Hall.

Berdes, C., and L. Emanuel. 2006. Adaptation in aging and dying: Ethical imperative or impossible dream? in *Death in the clinic*, ed. L. A. Jansen, 97–117. Lanham, MD: Rowman & Littlefield.

Brock, D. 1993. The ideal of shared decision making between patients and physicians. In *Life and death: Philosophical essays in biomedical ethics*, 21–54. New York: Cambridge University Press.

Callahan, D. 1993. Pursuing a peaceful death. *The Hastings Center Report* 23: 33–38.

CEJA. 1991. Council on Ethical and Judicial Affairs. Guidelines for the appropriate use of do-not-resuscitate orders. *JAMA* 265:1808–91.

CEJA. 1998–1999. Council on Ethical and Judicial Affairs. *Code of medical ethics: Current opinions*. Chicago: American Medical Association.

Emanuel, L. 1995. Structured deliberation to improve decision making for the seriously ill. *Hastings Center Report* 6:S14–S18.

Emanuel, L., and E. Emanuel. 1992. Four models of the doctor-patient relationship. *JAMA* 267:2221–26.

Field, M. J., and C. K. Cassell, eds. 1997. *Approaching death: Improving care at the end of life*. Washington, DC: National Academy Press.

Hallenbeck, J. L. 2000. Terminal sedation: Ethical implications in different situations. *Journal of Palliative Medicine* 3:313–20.

Jansen, L. A. 2006. Introduction. In *Death in the clinic*, ed. L. A. Jansen, 1–14. Lanham, MD: Rowman & Littlefield.

Jansen, L. A., B. Johnston, and D. P. Sulmasy. 2003. Ethical issues. In *A clinical guide to supportive and palliative care for HIV/AIDS*, ed. J. F. O'Neill, P. A. Selwyn, and H. Schietinger, 349–64. Washington, DC: U.S. Department of Health and Human Services.

Jansen, L. A., and D. P. Sulmasy. 2002. Proportionality, terminal sedation, and the restorative goals of medicine. *Theoretical Medicine and Bioethics* 23:321–37.

Kagan, S. 1989. *The limits of morality*. Oxford: Oxford University Press. See pp. 116–21.

Kamm, F. M. 1996. *Morality, mortality: Rights, duties, and status*. Vol. 2. Oxford: Oxford University Press.

Kant, I. 1964. *Groundwork of the metaphysics of morals*. Trans. H. J. Paton. New York: Harper and Row.

Lo, B., and G. Rubenfeld. 2005. Palliative sedation in dying patients: "We turn to it when everything else hasn't worked." *JAMA* 294:1810–16.

Quill, T. E., and H. Brody. 1996. Physician recommendations and patient autonomy: Finding a balance between physician power and patient choice. *Annals of Internal Medicine* 125(9): 763–69.

Quill, T. E., R. Dresser, and D. W. Brock. 1997a. The rule of double effect: A critique of its role at the end of life. *New England Journal of Medicine* 337:1768–71.

Quill, T. E., B. Lo, and D. W. Brock. 1997b. Palliative care options of the last resort: A comparison of voluntary stopping of eating and drinking, terminal sedation, physician assisted suicide, and voluntary active euthanasia. *JAMA* 278:2099–104.

Quill, T. E. and I. R. Byock. 2000. Responding to intractable terminal suffering: The role of terminal sedation and voluntary refusal of food and fluids. *Annals of Internal Medicine* 132: 400–14.

Quill, T. E., and D. E. Meier. 2006. The big chill—Inserting the DEA into end-of-life care. *New England Journal of Medicine* 354:1–3.

Schneiderman, L. J., N. Jecker, and A. Jonsen. 1990. Medical futility: Its meaning and ethical implications. *Annals of Internal Medicine* 112:949–54.

SUPPORT Study. 1995. A controlled trial to improve care for seriously ill hospitalized patients: The SUPPORT principle investigators. *JAMA* 274:1591–98.

Tomlinson, T., and D. Czlonka. 2000. Futility and hospital policy. In *Readings in health care ethics*, ed. E. Boetzkes and W. J. Waluchow, 419–29. Canada: Broadview Press.

Veatch, R. M. 1976. *Death, dying and the biological revolution: Our last quest for responsibility*. New Haven, CT: Yale University Press.

Velleman, D. J. 2006. Against the right to die. In *Death in the clinic*, ed. L. A. Jansen. Lanham, MD: Rowman & Littlefield.

9

Ethics in Pediatrics

Tracy K. Koogler

KEY POINTS

1. To explain the best interest standard and its importance in pediatric decision making.
2. To show how ethical decision making in pediatrics changes as the child becomes older.
3. To describe ways in which parents' decision making might be overridden by a hospital ethics committee (HEC) or physician.

When an HEC is requested to consult in pediatric cases, usually it occurs because of a conflict between the parents of a pediatric patient and the medical team. Typically, both parties believe that they have the child's best interests in mind and what is desired is for the consultation to resolve the conflict by making a clear decision about what is in the child's best interest. This can be a difficult position, because rarely is the decision as easy as one party being right and the other wrong. Since both parties have different relationships to the child, both are examining different interests of the child when determining best interests. With these differing perspectives on the same, usually complex situation, neither decision is completely right. This chapter, then, will begin by examining the "best interest" standard utilized in pediatrics in order to ground better our ethical decision making in the care of children. It will then focus on the role of and limits on parental refusal of treatments. Finally, it will look at some issues that arise at different developmental stages in childhood and adolescence.

BEST INTEREST STANDARD

Pediatric patients are different from adults in that they often lack decisional capacity to make medical decisions and have little to no experience in exercising decisional capacity generally, or specifically for making these kinds of decisions. It is for this reason that the best interest standard is utilized to make a decision for a child. That is, whereas "substituted judgment" should be employed where possible when making surrogate decisions for cognitively incapacitated adults who previously had decisional capacity, in the case of children (particularly very young children), to paraphrase Tristram Engelhardt (1996), we do not make decisions *with* them, but *for* them—typically they are unable to apply their own previously expressed interests (since those are rarely available, or even if available, rarely based on deep experience and careful consideration. More on the developmental character of children below). Instead, the best interest standard requires the decision maker to choose the option that is in the child's best interest and benefits the child, in light of the fact that the child is not, and has probably never been, well positioned to do this himself or herself. The question becomes who and what determine a child's best interests?

Unfortunately, no unanimity exists among ethicists. In general, following "best interests" requires that the child will benefit from the intervention and his or her overall welfare will be promoted, while avoiding unnecessary suffering. However, determining "benefit" and "overall welfare" is at the crux of the problem. On one side of the medical situation, the physicians and medical team aim to apply the best interest standard by presenting the medical options that they take to be in best interest of their pediatric patient. The parents, then, are expected to integrate the medically appropriate options into their sense of the familial and cultural interest of their child, with at least some attention to concerns for potential quality of life. It is precisely when parents choose an option that the physician does not see as in the child's best interest that ethical conflicts arise that can lead to HEC consultations. In many of these situations, the conflict revolves around a concern for quality of life as vital versus sanctity of life as paramount.

Ideally, we might want physicians only to examine medical indications when presenting care and treatment options to families; however, in reality, physicians often consider quality-of-life issues. This can be seen rather clearly when the child has (and will have) severe neurological limitation, with physicians more likely to recommend limitations of medical therapies because, in their estimation, the child either has a poor quality of life or will have a poor quality of life in the future (Burns et al. 2001). Of course, while some parents may come to a similar evaluation of their child's future quality of life, other parents may interpret their child's quality of life quite differently from the medical team's perception.

On the other side of the situation, children are usually members of families, and as such, family interests may weigh into the decision making of a parent when determining what is in a child's best interests. For example, a child's individual best interests may be served by allowing him to stay home and play; however, if his sister requires stitches, then he is likely to come to the hospital with the mother and sister so that her best interests are served. Of course, even here it can be argued that coming to the hospital with his mom and sister is in his best interest, since it keeps him safe from harm, under the protection of his mother. However, even this take acknowledges that the child and his specific interests do not live in isolation from, and are dependent on, others.

Traditionally, parents fulfill the role of decision maker for children, given their dependent and intimate relationship. Parents, in our society, are allowed a great deal of discretion in how they raise their children and are entitled to make educational, religious, and social decisions that affect their children. Parents incorporate family values into decision making for their children, which often involve consideration of a child's ethnic, religious, and personal backgrounds. However, with this deference to parental decision making comes many obligations to children to care for them, educate them, and provide food and shelter for them. So, while the parental right to make decisions for their children often goes unquestioned, it does so only as long as parents do not place the child in harm's way or in a life-threatening situation. Parents who are clearly harming or neglecting their children are often met with government intervention, through such channels as court orders of outside guardianship, custody by divisions of family and children services, or arrest by law enforcement.

Of course, parental decision making is a difficult task, and as noted above, parents must adjudicate the best interests of their child in light of many factors. While no child exists in isolation from dependence on others, and while the interests of others affected by the care of the child cannot be ignored in decision making, such interests can be difficult to weigh in light of the child's condition and needs. So, though parents routinely make decisions in the best interest of the family, it may not be in the best interests of an individual family member. When a child is ill, especially critically ill, the parents usually make decisions examining primarily, even exclusively, the child's best interests; however, in a few instances, family issues may play a more prominent role. For example, it is not unimportant to think about how the burden of care of this child may impact other children. A family might want palliative care for their child, but the thought of the child dying at home and potentially traumatizing other children is too difficult to implement.[1]

PARENTAL REFUSAL

As mentioned, parents are given a fair amount of latitude in making decisions for their children, so that they can raise them under their belief and value system. Given the variety of values and interests in the world, it is not surprising that parental beliefs and values can conflict with medicine's interpretation of a child's best interests. At these times, the physician, and in many situations HECs, must determine if the refusal of medical therapy is life threatening or significantly detrimental to that child. Legally, providing medically necessary treatments is required or otherwise may be considered parental abuse or neglect. Of course, the legal requirement only establishes concepts that require moral interpretation, and whether a family may be permitted to pursue an alternative form of therapy will depend greatly on the moral consideration of the situation at hand. Examples where concern might arise include: refusing immunizations, choosing an effective but not optimal medical treatment option, or pursuing herbal medical therapy for autism, and yet, for the most part, these parental decisions are legally, even morally, accepted. Medical professionals should respect the parents' rights to raise their children and preserve family values.

In situations in which there is substantial risk of serious harm to the child, however, the medical team must intervene (Diekema 2005). These situations might include the Jehovah's Witness parent who does not want his or her child who is bleeding profusely from a splenic laceration to obtain blood products, or the Christian Scientist parent who does not want antibiotics for his or her child with meningitis. These kinds of cases point out that parental decisions that are consistent with familial religious beliefs may not always be in the child's best interest to such a degree that it places the child in a life-threatening situation. While it is important to be sensitive to the fact that an important religious tenet with potentially extreme consequences exists, such as loss of heaven or banishment from the religious community, the best response to either situation above is to take legal protective custody of the children in order to provide them with appropriate medical therapy. It is settled case law in most states that the state has significant interest in protecting children, as potential contributors to society, in these conditions. The mechanism for taking protective custody in each state varies, and one should become familiar with one's state laws and procedures. In most states, the child will only be in temporary protective custody, and after the therapy is completed and the child is well, the child may return to the parents' custody.

The more difficult cases in this area involve uncertain prognoses, even with therapy, and situations in which the disease process will not be cured in a time-limited fashion. Take as an example a child with a brain tumor, who with therapy may have an additional six to twelve months of quality life but will ultimately die from his or her disease. If the parents refuse to bring the child to the hospital, should the child be removed from the home in order to obtain the therapy? What sense does it make to force the child to have therapy, against his or her parents' wishes, only to gain an additional six to twelve months? These are not easy decisions, and one must consider the age and cognitive awareness of the child, especially if he or she is old enough to understand the situation. Aggressive action to force therapy with which the child's parents disagree may make him or her quite distraught, especially if there is a religious basis.

Decisions in the gray area are difficult and time consuming. Many times, trying to give the parents time to adjust to the diagnosis and evaluate the therapy is helpful. Parents' initial "no" may simply mean,

"I am too overwhelmed with the diagnosis and prognosis to make any decisions now."

Further, cases in which the child is diagnosed with a chronic disease often prove the most difficult. For instance, take a practicing Christian Scientist whose child is diagnosed with type 1 diabetes. On the one hand, medical indications tell us that without insulin, this child will die; on the other hand, church doctrine states that everything can be healed through prayer. Here, again, significant values are at stake, with the health, well-being, and even life of a child in the balance. If the conflict proves intractable, the case often results in the child being taken from the home and placed in foster care. Such an outcome is unfortunate, even tragic. Many, if not all, parents in these situations dearly love their children and want what is best for them, and yet it is precisely the conflict between medical indications and spiritual values that makes determining what is best so difficult. As a society, we have decided that children who are *not yet* able maturely to hold the values of their parents (and others) *as their own* should not be subjected to potential harm because of them (this becomes even more challenging as children mature into adolescence). Thus, court intervention can become necessary.

To be clear, though, as HEC members pondering these cases, one must remember that requiring medical therapy without parental consent entails going against the family's values and sometimes religious tenets. Although, as individuals, we may not agree or understand their values, we must respect their values just as we would want our personal and religious values to be respected. Therefore, court-ordered therapy should only be done in situations in which it is clear that the therapy will be life prolonging or life preserving. Though watching the Jehovah's Witness child with the low hematocrit can be difficult, in an attempt to respect the family's religious beliefs, with the hemodynamically stable child, it is best to watch and wait.

SPECIFIC ISSUES WITHIN AGE GROUPS

As we have begun to see in situations of parental refusal, the developmental stages of the child also affect decision making, because although children under the age of eighteen years, in general, do not have the legal right to make medical decisions (see section on teens for exceptions), children clearly may express an opinion about certain decisions as they grow older. In general, the one-year-old who screams in seeming protest at the time of his or her immunizations has his or her protests largely ignored, though the child is comforted after the fact. However, the school-age child may be given a choice between pills and liquid medication, or even perhaps when semielective surgery is to be done, this week or next month, during school vacation. The teenager is beginning to develop complex decision-making skills and may have clear ideas about his or her medical care, especially if he or she has been living with a disease for a long period of time. Thus, we will examine some issues that arise at different developmental stages.

NEWBORNS

The newborn period is unique because decisions are made about patients who have no history with a family and in which their entire life is before them. For infants born significantly premature (twenty-two to twenty-four weeks), as well as infants with severe birth defects, such as Trisomy 13 or 18, or anencephaly, complex decision making begins in the delivery room, where families may have to consider the options whether to approach treatment options aggressively or even to resuscitate. Often, this decision making is a joint process between the neonatologist and the parents; however, in some situations, the institution (by policy) or neonatologist (by practice) may decide that aggressive care is unwarranted—based on the severity of the condition or the extreme degree of prematurity.

Reasons for these policies and practices in medicine vary. In some cases, neonatologists base their considerations on medical findings where research shows that very premature infants (twenty-three weeks and younger) or with extremely low birth weights (500 grams or less) are difficult to resuscitate and even if resuscitated, have poor long-term survival (Vohr and Allen 2005). Of course, these kinds of findings are targeted on mortality. However, in other cases such as Trisomy 13 and 18, in which the child is certain to have significant neurological delays, some physicians focus on quality-of-life considerations advocating for comfort measures, rather than aggressive, curative treatment attempts. Traditionally, physicians have considered such neurological and chromosomal conditions to be lethal anomalies, with children dying before a year of age despite therapy. Recently, with some families questioning physicians and demanding more aggressive medical and surgical therapies for these children, some have lived beyond a year of age, and even a few children survive into their early teens (Baty 1994). It is important to note that the degree of developmental delay is significant, with most children being nonverbal, unable to walk or even crawl, and only able to function at the level of an infant. However, some parents have been able to incorporate these children into their families, enjoy their lives, and believe these children possess an acceptable quality of life.

While the extreme cases can place physicians and parents on different sides, with parents desiring treatments that physicians think inappropriate, occasionally, the roles can be reversed. Paradigmatic are those situations where an infant's level of maturity (twenty-six to twenty-eight weeks or beyond) or disorder (for example, Trisomy 21) makes the medical team feel obligated to provide aggressive treatments and resuscitation while the parents state a preference to forego such actions. These parents often request comfort measures, but the reasons for their request can be as much about fear of developmental disabilities, especially with a premature infant, as they are about medical facts. Although many former premature infants have only mild delays (Mikkola et al. 2005), parents may see the prematurity, prolonged hospitalization, and probable developmental delay as too great a burden for the child and family. In such cases, emotional burdens will be great. While ethically appropriate, most parents find it more difficult to withdraw the ventilator once it has been instituted than to ask for the child to be wrapped in a blanket and placed in the parents' arms at the time of delivery. And yet, most neonatologists beyond a certain gestation—twenty-four to twenty-six weeks—want to resuscitate initially (American Heart Association 2005). Often the compromise position is to provide initial medical support for the infant but stop aggressive therapy should the child be found to have significant neurological injury from intracranial bleeds or other overly burdensome anomalies.

One last turn are those situations in which a parent wants to withhold or withdraw therapy on a term infant with genetic abnormalities that result in developmental delay. Specific discussion of such cases has an interesting history. In the 1970s, Duff and Campbell (1973) wrote about intentionally not being aggressive with these infants and not performing life-saving surgeries on these children so that they could be permitted to die. By the 1980s, the public had become concerned that infants with Trisomy 21, and other forms of developmental delay, were being allowed to die from *treatable* medical conditions such as tracheoesophageal fistulas and simple heart defects.

After several attempts at regulation (Baby Doe regulations of the U.S. Department of Health and Human Services [DHHS]), this concern led to the federal government passing regulations as amendments to the 1984 Child Abuse Prevention and Treatment Act (a.k.a. the Child Abuse Amendments; see DHHS 1982, 1983, 1984). The regulations required states to develop a process by which to respond to cases of nontreatment of handicapped newborns, leading most physicians to become more aggressive in their medical management of mentally and physically handicapped newborns so that they would not be accused of discrimination. These regulations have a narrow list of exceptions, including: (a) if the infant is chronically and irreversibly comatose; (b) if the provision of such treatment would (i) merely prolong dying, (ii) not be effective in ameliorating or correcting all the infant's life-threatening conditions, or (iii) otherwise be futile in terms of the survival of the infant; or (c) if the provision of such treatment would be virtually futile or inhumane. The regulations specified that anencephaly met the second criteria, but it remains uncertain if other devastating birth defects such as Trisomy 13 and 18 clearly meet the definitions (DHHS 1982, 1983, 1984).

As noted above, neonatologists will support and even recommend comfort measures only for some of these disorders, such as anencephaly and Trisomy 18, while mandating therapy for others, such as Trisomy 21 and spina bifida. Other disorders, for example, hypoplastic left-heart syndrome, continue to be in a gray zone, in which some physicians and institutions would recommend no aggressive therapy and others would mandate therapy.

DEVELOPING THROUGH CHILDHOOD AND GAINING ASSENT

Except in some significant cases, as children grow, so do their levels of experience and intelligence. As such, medical decision making about pediatric patients affects children who become cognizant of the issues, treatments, demands, and concerns—to varying degrees, of course. As such, including children in the medical decision-making process becomes more and more important as the child grows.

Assent is a concept that allows the child who has some basic understanding of a situation to agree or assent to a procedure. As endorsed by the American Academy of Pediatrics (AAP) Committee on Bioethics (1995), pediatricians should be aware of a developmental-staged approach to assent with their patients.[2] The AAP guidelines state that for the most part, children under the age of seven may be told about possible treatments, but their participation in decision making is unnecessary. However, in children over seven years of age, it is recommended that physicians gain a child's assent before a procedure. This requires that the physician explain to the patient in an understandable fashion what is proposed and why, gaining his or her agreement to the proposal. While this may be the standard for caring for school-age children, in practice, it can be much more difficult. In practice, what would and should happen if assent is not obtained? What level of treatment would cease without assent? For example, it would seem difficult to justify stopping, or even delaying, necessary medical therapy to a young child because she or he does not want it because it may hurt or be inconvenient. Would the same hold for a routine shot or even bad-tasting medications?

Of course, this raises a serious question about the status of "assent" in pediatric care. In practice, is assent only to be respected when the child, in fact, agrees to the proposed course of treatment? Does "assent" not imply that a child is entitled to "dissent" as well? If not, what function does the assent process truly serve? Unless there is substantive agreement that the assent process involves a genuine choice for the patient, it would seem we only need to require that the physician explain the situation, answer any questions, and provide any allowances in the medical therapy that the child might actually get to determine—for example, which arm to try first for an IV or which flavor to smell when one is being anesthetized for a procedure.

TEENAGERS

As children develop to adolescence, new ethical challenges arise. Teens begin to emerge as complex decision makers, and some teens are capable of thoughtfully considering medical options. For this reason, the concept of the mature minor has developed. The AAP suggests that adolescent teens, usually over the age of fourteen, who are thoughtful about the medical issues should be encouraged to express their interests pertaining to medical care and, at times, even make the primary medical decision. Having said this, whether such a mature minor would be legally allowed to consent is a matter of individual state law. As a legal matter, it is not enough to assume that any particular state does or does not allow legal consent from a minor (who meets certain conditions), since these issues vary state by state.

Regardless of the particular legal issues, however, certain ethical standards should apply. First, teens should be included in the conversations about their medical therapies. Diagnoses and reasonable medical options should be discussed with them. This can prove difficult for parents who may be fearful of upsetting their child, and yet, unlike the neonate or toddler, respecting the maturing teen requires that we not just act on them, but with them. The mature minor should be encouraged to participate in his or her care, expressing opinions that are respected by the medical team. While parents may retain the legal right to consent to medical treatment, they should be reminded that their child is aware of and able to understand what is going on around him or her and, therefore, should be actively included. A real danger arises when parents try to exclude teens from difficult decisions, in an attempt to protect them, as this can result in making the teen angry, resentful, and alienated from the parents. Such consequences are tragic given that some patients find themselves at a time when they most need family support and comfort.

Of course, encouraging participation in the decision-making process can result in a teenage patient who, in fact, declines particular therapies. Possibly the most challenging of these situations arises when a mature minor wants to refuse ongoing life-saving therapy in order to be allowed to die. With certain chronic conditions, the teen and parents may have dramatically different views on how the illness should be managed in the end stages. For example, the parents of the child with Duchenne's muscular dystrophy (DMD) may desire chronic mechanical ventilation and full resuscitative attempts, while their son may believe that it is time to cease such aggressive efforts so that he be allowed to die. Experience in the son's life may inform his decision, experience the parents do not have intimate access to. If their son attends camp for children with DMD, he may have noticed that his friends are not coming back each year, and he realizes they have died. He may also have seen kids who have opted for mechanical ventilation. While these kinds of experiences lead him to the idea that he would not want to be kept alive on machines, his parents may not understand—desiring instead that his life be prolonged as long as possible. Such conflicts demonstrate the persistent difficulty in ethical decision making, as both parties express good reasons for their wishes. Each side is concerned for the well-being of the patient, with the teen himself able to connect his desires to a reasonable account of his experiences, while the parents' love and care for their child is evident in their desire to keep him alive. Such decisions rarely lend themselves to an easy fix, and multiple discussions should occur before any decisions are made. All invested parties should have an opportunity to voice their opinions, and everyone should listen to those opinions and be respectful. In these cases, HEC consults rely heavily on mediation and facilitation skills so that a decision can be reached, one that hopefully satisfies all interested parties.

However, not all refusals are thoughtful. Teens are still maturing and, as such, are prone to "magical" thinking that prevents them from acknowledging critical illness, especially when it is of a chronic nature. Such thinking leads to life-threatening behaviors with teens not taking medications or following treatment protocols—for example, avoiding taking insulin for the diabetic, bronchodilators for the asthmatic, or immunosuppressives for the transplant patient. Adherence to chronic therapy regimens is not simply useful, it can be vital. Nonadherence, then, becomes a very difficult issue to work through for healthcare providers. On the one hand, medical personnel recognize that parents are trying to give their maturing children both some freedoms and also some responsibilities concerning their illnesses and medications. On the other hand, when the child is placed in charge of his or her own therapy and does not adhere to the regimen, the parents may be seen as neglectful, and in fact, may be neglectful. Parents should be cautioned against allowing their child's medical habits to go unchecked, monitoring such behaviors just as one might stay on top of large homework assignments and curfews. In fact, these behaviors can have consequences for later medical decisions, such as in issues of retransplanting a child who has rejected his or her organ. Whether another transplant is warranted may turn on the basis of nonadherence. State intervention may follow if the family is considered dangerously neglectful.

Whether participants to their care, accepting, rejecting, even nonadhering to treatment plans, teenagers are a challenging class of patients, since so much of our ethic in medicine is based on the fully mature, autonomous adult or the completely cognitively immature infant. Even the law recognizes the difficulty, with some states allowing mature minors of sufficient intelligence to make their own medical decisions and other states not. However, in most every state there are special circumstances under which teenagers can make their own medical decisions, even when a specific mature minor clause does not exist.

In most states, teenagers may become "emancipated." This is a special legal circumstance in which a minor under the age of eighteen becomes legally independent from his or her parents. Emancipation either occurs because of marriage or requires a court decision, and the teen must be living on his or her own and providing his or her own income. Further, teens who are pregnant or are already parents may be treated in some states as emancipated to make decisions for themselves, or simply be treated as the legal decision maker for their children. As with mature minor clauses, emancipation laws vary state to state. It is important for HEC members to have access to good legal advice in order to know how or if state laws apply in a particular case.

Another special circumstance in which a teen may be able to seek out and receive medical therapy without parental consent is with regard to sexual issues, psychological issues, and substance use issues. The goal of these exceptions is to encourage teens to receive necessary medical care without fear of parental notification. Ethically, these exceptions often raise important concerns for confidentiality, especially when pediatricians have long-term relationships with parents as well as children. Pediatricians may be conflicted when the parent asks the physician to explore areas of sexuality or substance use. Alternatively, the medical professional himself or herself may feel it important to disclose information to parents in order to improve a child's safety or compliance with medical therapy. In either case, discussion should occur with the teen about the advantages and risks of discussing the issue with the parents, offering different ways to talk with the parents— for example, the teen can discuss alone, the healthcare professional can speak to the parents, or the teen and the healthcare provider can talk to the parents together. If the teen is uncomfortable with all of these options, then it is advisable to respect his or her choice but continue conversations so that one might support the child in crisis and also find a way to get him or her support from home.

Finally, though parents often have the right to make medical decisions for teenagers, parents cannot *demand* certain medical tests, such as drug screening, pregnancy tests, and so forth, without the teenager's knowledge and assent. Exceptions may be made for medical reasons when the practitioner deems the testing necessary in extraordinary circumstances—for example, the child is comatose and has symptoms of an overdose, or the girl has abdominal pain and bleeding. Again, negotiations can occur with the parents, teen, and the healthcare practitioner, and openness and honesty must be maintained throughout. The balance to be maintained remains between allowing the teen to have some control over his or her body and protecting the teen against foolish decisions that will regrettably threaten health and welfare.

CONCLUSION

Pediatric ethical decision making is based on the principle of best interests of the child, with a concern for patient autonomy growing as the child develops maturity and intelligence. In most cases, parents are afforded the legal right to be the primary decision maker for their children until children are eighteen years of age. Parents are the appropriate decision makers who will bring issues of quality of life and familial values into the decision-making process, while healthcare professionals should present the medically appropriate options and allow the family to determine how those options fit with familial values and best support an acceptable quality of life.

The developmental stages of childhood affect how the medical team should interact with the child in the decision-making process. Children under the age of seven are usually told what will happen to them, but we are unlikely to take their protests against an unpleasant experience necessary to treat or diagnose a medical condition as determinative. Children between seven and fourteen may be able to give assent to a procedure, and yet, depending on the severity of the condition or vital importance of treatment, their decision may be overruled. The teenager over the age of fourteen is developing complex decision-making skills and should be included in discussions of healthcare options. Respect for teens' perspectives and incorporation of their thoughts into the medical care plan is preferred whenever possible, and due deference to their desires should be paid.

FOR FURTHER REFLECTION

1. A sixteen-year-old boy has lymphoma with a 90-percent survival rate with chemotherapy. His parents do not want him to be treated for religious reasons. What do you do as the HEC consultant? Does the child's opinion about therapy matter, that is, he either agrees or disagrees with his parents' decision?

2. An infant is born with Trisomy 21 (Down syndrome) and tetralogy of fallot (complex congenital heart disease), which requires surgery in the first week of life and probably subsequent surgeries. The parents do not want to consent to surgery and want to take the child home with palliative care. What do you do as the HEC consultant?

NOTES

1. There is some debate about the role of familial interests when determining the "best interests" of a child. While Buchanan and Brock (1989) argue for a singular focus on "self regarding interests" of the child, I take Lainie Ross's (1998) position that familial interest must have some role in that determination. See Allen Buchanan and Dan Brock, *Deciding for Others: The Ethics of Surrogate Decision Making* (Oxford University Press, 1989) and Lainie Friedman Ross, *Children, Families, and Health Care Decision Making* (Oxford University Press, 1998).

2. A recent study has shown that few physicians are aware of and applying the guidelines. Lee K. J., Havens P. L., Sato T. T., Hoffman G. M., Leuthner S. R. 2006. "Assent for Treatment: Clinician Knowledge, Attitudes, and Practice. *Pediatrics* (2): 723–30.

WORKS CITED

American Academy of Pediatrics, Committee on Bioethics. 1995. Informed consent, parental permission, and assent in pediatric practice. *Pediatrics* 95: 314.

American Heart Association. 2005. 2005 American Heart Association (AHA) guidelines for cardiopulmonary resuscitation (CPR) and emergency cardiovascular care (ECC) of pediatric and neonatal patients: Pediatric basic life support. *Circulation* 112 (24): suppl. IV1–203.

Baty, B. J. 1994. Natural history of Trisomy 18 and Trisomy 13: I. Growth, physical assessment, medical histories, survival, and recurrance risk. *American Journal of Medical Genetics* 49 (2): 175–88.

Burns, J. P., C. Mitchell, J. L. Griffith, and R. D. Truog. 2001. End-of-life care in the pediatric intensive care unit: Attitudes and practices of pediatric critical care physicians and nurses. *Critical Care Medicine* 29 (3): 658–64.

DHHS. Department of Health and Human Services. 1982. Notice to health care providers: Discriminating against handicapped by withholding treatment or nourishment. *Federal Register* 47, no. 116 (June 16, 1982): 26027.

———. 1983. Interim final rule. Nondiscrimination on the basis of handicap relating to health care for handicapped infants. *Federal Register* 48, no. 45 (July 5, 1983): 30846.

———. 1984. Final rule. Nondiscrimination on the basis of handicap: Procedures and guidelines relating to health care for handicapped infants. *Federal Register* 49, no. 8 (January 12, 1984).

Diekema, D. S. 2005. Responding to parental refusals of immunizations. *Pediatrics* 115 (5): 1428–31.

Duff, R. S., and A. G. M. Campbell. 1973. Moral and ethical dilemmas in the special care nursery. *New England Journal of Medicine* 289:890–94.

Englehardt, H. T. 1996. *The foundations of bioethics.* New York: Oxford University Press.

Mikkola, K., N. Ritari, V. Tommiska, et al. 2005. Neurodevelopmental outcome at 5 years of age of a national cohort of extremely low birth weight infants who were born in 1996–1997. *Pediatrics* 116 (6): 1391–400.

Vohr, B. R., and M. Allen. 2005. Extreme prematurity—The continuing dilemma. *New England Journal of Medicine* 352 (1): 71–72.

10

The Hospital Ethics Committee as Educator

Kathy Kinlaw

KEY POINTS

1. Assess the ethics knowledge level at your organization.
2. Education of hospital ethics committee (HEC) members is intertwined with the education of the full organizational staff.
3. Recognize the practical moral wisdom and expertise of colleagues at your institution.
4. The process of education matters—it should be highly relevant and engaging, utilize existing forums, and use multiple educational methodologies.
5. Acknowledge the complexity of ethics in action.
6. Track and evaluate HEC's educational efforts.

Of all of the potential roles of HECs, the role of "educator" is arguably the most fundamental and enduring role of the committee. In addition to traditional training opportunities, every policy examined, every retrospective review of a recurring issue at the hospital, every organizational and managed-care issue studied, and every concurrent consultation becomes an opportunity for education—not only for committee members but also for patients, families, and the hospital staff at large. An effective HEC will consider carefully and intentionally how its role as educator will be articulated and implemented and how the institution will evaluate the committee's effectiveness in this role.

PRELIMINARY QUESTIONS FOR YOUR INSTITUTION

In order to target education appropriately, certain foundational assessment questions must be addressed before the HEC can take on the role of educator.

Does the hospital staff even know that an HEC exists or is being formed at the hospital?

Early in the life of an HEC or at a critical juncture for assessing the work of an existing HEC, surveying hospital physicians and other staff members is a powerful tool. The first question for such a survey might be "Is there an HEC at 'X' hospital?" Responses of "yes," "no," and "unsure" provide quick information about the level of awareness of the HEC. A follow-up question addressing "If so, which of the following are roles of the HEC at 'X?'" will also provide further information both about respondent understanding *and* the effectiveness of the HEC in communicating its roles.

Does the staff know what an ethics committee is and is not?

Education is not the role most closely associated with most ethics committees, and yet the task of education by the HEC is essential to the committee's ability to perform its other roles. Many healthcare professionals, when asked what ethics committees actually do, think first of the HEC as providing consultation in difficult cases. For some professionals, this consulting role is misperceived as one of monitoring and oversight of decision making. This perceived "second guessing" of traditional healthcare decision making along with concerns about the preparedness and effectiveness of committees as consultants raise concerns for many physicians. Physician-ethicist Mark Siegler warned about the potential for ethics committees to undermine the physician/patient relationship by interrupting the physician's authority in decision making (Siegler 1986). The demythologizing of ethics committee consultation is being addressed in other chapters of this book (see chapters 4 and 5), but an early task for ethics committees *as educators* is to recognize this potential suspicion and mistrust and to address it proactively throughout the hospital. A survey mechanism developed to get at the prevailing knowledge about and attitudes toward the HEC can aid in addressing the issues, interests, and concerns of the hospital staff.

HEC SELF-EDUCATION

In order for the HEC to provide effective ethics education to the hospital staff, ethics committee members themselves must have adequate ethics education. Committees should include, therefore, members with ethics expertise or should have ethics resource people readily available. Additionally, HEC members must identify effective *mechanisms* for self-education and develop a basic understanding of the field of clinical and organizational ethics themselves. According to a University of Pennsylvania survey of HEC chairs from 1998 to 1999, HECs do spend a significant percentage of time in self-education. Of the 322 responding hospitals with an HEC, chairs reported that the mean amount of time spent on HEC self-education was 29.8 percent. In fact, this activity constituted the largest percentage of reporting HECs' time (McGee et al. 2001).[1]

Self-education of ethics committee members prepares committee members with skills to contribute effectively to all of the functions of the HEC—education, consultation, policy review and formulation, and evaluation. The areas of expertise needed for case consultation as identified in the American Society for Bioethics and Humanities' (ASBH's) core competencies for consultation in 1998 are relevant for HEC self-education (see Table 10.1).

This document recognizes that there are some areas in which all HEC members should have basic knowledge or skill and other areas in which advanced knowledge or skill is needed. While this advanced knowledge or skill may not be possessed by all members of an HEC,

---

Table 10.1.   American Society for Bioethics and Humanities' Core Knowledge Areas for Ethics Consultation

1. Moral reasoning and ethical theory
2. Bioethical issues and concepts that typically emerge
3. Healthcare systems including managed care and governmental systems
4. Clinical context, such as medical terminology, common diseases, and emerging technologies
5. Healthcare institution in which consultants work, including institutional policies
6. Beliefs and perspectives of patient and staff population served by organization
7. Relevant codes of ethics, professional conduct, and accrediting organizations' guidelines
8. Relevant health law

at least one member of an HEC should have expertise in each area, or someone who has this background should be available to the committee through external resources (ASBH 1998). In order for the HEC to participate effectively in educating the broader hospital staff, a reasonable level of HEC members' understanding about the scope of clinical and organizational ethics is necessary.

In order to target HEC self-education forums, it is good practice to survey HEC members routinely about areas in which they desire additional ethics education as well as those areas where their knowledge and comfort is highest. In conjunction with such needs assessments, it is also good practice to survey HEC members in order to identify areas of expertise or interest in providing committee or staff education. All HEC members have certain areas of expertise and experience that may provide powerful foundations for education. For example, an HEC member who is a hospice nurse can bring both patient narratives and questions around the ethics of end-of-life care to educational forums; a transplant surgeon can raise ethical questions about transplant selection criteria and where issues of patient ability to adhere to posttransplant care intersect with concerns about equity and fairness. If there is an HEC member who is a risk manager, she or he can richly discuss patient care concerns around the ethics of disclosure of medical error. Every HEC should look at its own membership for areas of expertise. Pairing these area experts with a clinical ethicist may provide the basis for a highly relevant educational discussion, even early in the HEC member's tenure. When area experts become increasingly informed about ethics as a discipline, the HEC member can effectively provide education on his or her own.

ENABLING THE HEC AS EDUCATOR

Several factors facilitate the ability of the membership of an ethics committee to serve as a resource for a hospital. Of paramount importance is support of hospital leadership in communicating the importance of ethics. Further, members (and their supervisors) must recognize that HEC membership will require a commitment to learning about the field of ethics and a significant time commitment, quite different from many other hospital committees. In order for committees to effectively bring a body of expertise to education, members must be willing to learn about the normative approaches to ethics in addition to bringing their rich experiences and their understanding of professional virtue.

Acknowledging the "practical moral wisdom" (or *phronesis*) that most healthcare professionals possess (Churchill and Schenck 2005) is important for both HEC members as well as those hospital colleagues on which educational programs are focused. Ethical reflection builds upon these strengths and provides additional ways of framing issues and thus should serve as a resource, rather than be viewed as a critiquing rival. HEC education should both support the traditional physician/health team/patient/family relationship as the locus of decision making and be highly relevant to those physician and hospital staff members on the front line. Helping physician and hospital staff members examine and clarify their own ethical values, beliefs, and decision-making styles provides a basis for thoughtful, more impartial examination of ethical issues.

PERCEIVED RELEVANCE

As mentioned above, relevance of HEC education can be strengthened by utilizing a hospital-wide survey mechanism. Physician and hospital staff members can assess the frequency with which particular clinical, research, or organizational issues occur and the degree to which these issues are viewed as ethically problematic. Analysis of responses according to demographic information—such as across and within professional disciplines or by affected patient care floors or units—provides important information about what issues may be recurrent and whether issues are discipline- or unit-specific. These indicators provide information that can shape the way in which relevant ethics education proceeds in the institution.

While HEC members will need to develop a foundational level of understanding in a broad array of contemporary ethical topics, educational programming for the broader hospital staff must be focused. Selecting a recurring issue or a topic surfaced by a recent difficult clinical case or organizational issue ensures a level of interest. Additionally, addressing a cutting-edge issue or one that has had recent national attention may help colleagues stay up to date and challenged in their thinking. (See Table 10.2.)

Table 10.2.   Sample Topics for Ethics Education of Physician and Hospital Staff

- Withdrawal of Artificial Hydration and Nutrition: Lessons Learned from the Story of Terri Schiavo
- Altered Medical Standards: Whether and When Emergent Conditions Justify a Different Level of Treatment
- Ethical Issues in Genetics and Predictive Health
- Legal and Ethical Perspectives on Decision Making near the End of Life (multiple program topics: advance directives, DNR decisions, withholding and withdrawal of treatment, the question of medical futility, brain death, organ transplantation, assisted suicide)
- Access to Health Care for Illegal Immigrants
- Ethical Issues in Pandemic Influenza
- Neuroethics
- Patient Confidentiality, Privacy, and Respect in the HIPAA Era
- Respecting Difference: How are Ethical Issues Framed and by Whom? (a nuanced look at whether and how race, ethnicity, culture, religion, alternative understandings of illness, family systems, and other perspectives unique to those involved in a case make a difference)
- The Evolving Ethics of Life's Start (reproductive technologies, fetal surgery, personhood, neonatal ethics)
- Access, Equity of Care, and the Long-term Survival of Health Systems

---

Ethics education formats may be most effective when healthcare professionals are first engaged through mechanisms that focus on relevance or practice impact, followed by utilizing the language of ethics to clarify, reframe, or analyze the practice question. Thus, the case study approach is a frequent mechanism in ethics education. Context-rich, detailed narratives of real cases, preferably from the organization's own experience, provide a compelling entry point for frontline professionals. Additional, engaging mechanisms include: mock ethics committee meetings in which exploration of an issue and the communication issues embedded in the discussion are demonstrated; utilization of simulated patient encounters with actors or scripted HEC members playing particular roles; watching a video or portion of a commercial film in which an issue is illustrated; or, in the right small-group setting, reading a short story or theater script. Each of these mechanisms provides a powerful experience, but its effectiveness in ethics education necessitates that it is accompanied by a well-moderated discussion of the ethical issues illustrated along with clear teaching points.

THE COMPLEXITY OF ETHICAL ACTION

In addition to addressing relevant practice issues, HECs have an opportunity to help physician and hospital staff members understand the process of ethical engagement. Case consultation methodologies (see chapter 4), which are helpful in analyzing specific cases, are only one part of the process of promoting ethical action. Understanding the broader context of how ethical action evolves may be very helpful for HECs. One model for ethical action is derived from the work of educational psychologist James Rest (Rest and Narvaez 1994). This model identifies four components as essential to ethical action:

1. **Ethical sensitivity or attentiveness**, which incorporates the ability both to recognize that the issue is an ethical one (rather than primarily a legal issue or a cultural issue or a scientific/ medical issue, and so on) and to acknowledge one's role responsibility or "agency" in addressing it.
2. **Ethical reasoning**, which invites one to carefully analyze the situation utilizing various normative approaches and theories (such as those addressed in chapter 3 herein).
3. **Ethical commitment**, which examines one's willingness to act, based on the acknowledgment of other, very real, competing commitments, often of a nonmoral nature (time, self-preservation, conflict avoidance, and so forth).
4. **Ethical character/implementation**, which assesses whether one will actually take the next steps and knows what resources and practical options exist in order to move forward.

Rest and Narvaez (1994) indicate that all four of these components must be present for ethical action to occur. This model acknowledges that ethical issues are situated in complex contexts, and awareness of these layers and practice competencies may be powerful for medical and hospital staffs. Before one can analyze a situation, one must be able to recognize what ethical issues are at stake. Such recognition and naming is rarely a simple task; multiple involved parties may provide varying perspectives on what they believe is at stake. Once identified ethical issues are carefully analyzed, one still must decide whether one will actually speak up or act in the complexity of a situation where action has consequences and skills are needed to move the issue forward effectively. Healthcare professionals can resonate with what is at stake in the midst of difficult decisions.

ACKNOWLEDGING EXISTING EDUCATIONAL PATTERNS

Logistics also matter in constructing educational opportunities, and existing forums provide important venues for ethics education. Each hospital unit has existing administrative and educational meetings. If ICU staff meetings occur at a weekly time, working with meeting conveners to address an ethics issue at this existing meeting—perhaps somewhat extended—may best respect that staff's time and result in well-attended discussions. The ethics session may need to be repeated during other shifts. HEC members can work with unit leaders to determine a topic of current interest or concern (Is a new ethics-related policy being implemented in the hospital or unit? Did unit staff struggle with a difficult patient case recently? Are there recurring ethical issues in the unit that staff would like to address?).

Each meeting provides a challenge to see if ethics is relevant to the everyday life of staff, patients, and families. Some issues can best be addressed in a discussion format in which procedural ethics is modeled as unit staff are able to voice their concerns and questions that help frame the ethical issues are asked. Because limited time is available in existing forums, especially when other agenda items are also addressed, HEC members' initial discussions may lead to an invitation to return for a more in-depth dialogue. Simply the presence of the HEC members and their method of approaching the discussion will convey important information about the overall role and effectiveness of the HEC.

Further, which members of the HEC lead the educational forum (and why *these* members) should be carefully addressed. An HEC member who is knowledgeable about the practices of a particular unit may be especially helpful in the discussion, but only if staff in that unit can acknowledge that in this discussion, the individual has a separate role as a member of the HEC and possesses a level of expertise in ethics. Additionally, seeing the discussion through, including subsequent meetings, and following up with participants and unit spokespeople will be important to determining the functional role of the HEC within the hospital.

OTHER OPPORTUNITIES FOR ETHICS EDUCATION

Beyond existing divisional and unit meetings, there may be other opportunities for education organization-wide. Medical staff meetings or Grand Round formats provide collaborative opportunities to address large groups who are already accustomed to attending the forum. Creating separate ethics grand rounds may work in some organizational settings.

Additionally, bringing ethical discussions to leadership groups (such as the medical executive committee or conflict of interest committee or the hospital board) may provide an important resource for these groups and will demonstrate the importance of the work of the HEC as a resource to the organization. Having members of these leadership groups also serve on the membership of the HEC provides an ongoing mechanism for information exchange and assists in the identification of issues about which the HEC might provide further education. Where other hospital committees have responsibilities that clearly intersect with ethical concerns in the organization, HECs should establish regular mechanisms for discussion and information sharing. Risk management committees, institutional research boards, compliance programs, and separate organizational ethics committees provide important collaborators for impacting ethical issues systemwide.

Finally, nontraditional strategies for education can also be important for HECs to consider. For example:

- The practice of including ethics as a part of new staff orientation identifies clearly the importance of ethics at an organization. At this level, basic information may be most helpful: what do we mean by ethics and why is it important; respect for differing values of patients, visitors, and colleagues; and information on the role of the HEC and how to access it. Making ethical questions engaging and relevant will be important to the success of including ethics in orientation programs.
- A brochure and posted announcements that describe the purpose of the HEC and how to access it as a resource may help colleagues (and patients and visitors) begin to understand the role of the HEC.
- Inclusion of timely ethical articles in hospital staff newsletters, on websites, or via other established communication routes provides an opportunity for more in-depth coverage of issues.

- Every note that an HEC team or member writes in the chart becomes an educational tool for anyone accessing the chart.

ACCOUNTABILITY AND EFFECTIVENESS

Evaluation of the effectiveness of the HEC in achieving each of its stated roles and responsibilities is essential. HECs should utilize outcomes research resources at the organization in determining a methodology for assessing whether it has been effective in providing education to healthcare colleagues. Utilizing the survey tool discussed earlier would provide a baseline about knowledge level and areas of interest. HECs can track their educational activities throughout the year and describe such meeting information as number, frequency, format, topic, and attendees. In addition, participants could provide brief meeting evaluations providing quick responses about attendee satisfaction, knowledge gained, likelihood of changing behavior, effectiveness of presenters and formats, and identification of future topics of interest. In some settings, pre- and post-tests can be utilized to better assess the knowledge and skills gained. It would also be helpful to initiate periodic follow-up assessments with clinicians who have participated in educational programming to determine whether and how the information gained had impacted their practice. Similarly, soliciting feedback from individuals involved in more informal educational formats (for example, monthly meetings with the risk management committee) may provide valuable evaluative information. Because each consultation is also an opportunity for education, follow-up questionnaires with those involved in case consultation also provides significant information about knowledge gained. A year-end, organization-wide survey covering those knowledge and skill areas that were the focus of that year's educational programming, would provide an assessment of community understanding along with direction for future programming opportunities.

HEC AS EDUCATOR

HECs are not alone in serving as ethics educators in their communities. Many regions have an ethics consortium or collaborative that provides educational programming for interested healthcare professionals and can supplement and support HECs in their role as educators. National educational programming is available through university-based bioethics centers, professional associations, and national associations like the ASBH. HECs can make information about these broader programs available to physician and hospital staff members. Yet, given the constraints on healthcare professionals' time and institutional resources, educational opportunities "at home" within the organization may be the most effective way for healthcare professionals to address ethical issues and for ethical reflection to permeate organizational culture. HEC leadership and members should remain keenly aware that all HEC actions and responsibilities become "ethics teaching moments" for colleagues. Tracking educational activity and impact provides important information about the effectiveness of the HEC for organizational leadership and the organization as a whole.

FOR FURTHER REFLECTION

1. What mechanisms would allow your HEC to assess the ethics knowledge level at your organization, and what resources and institutional support do you need to make this assessment possible?
2. What are the primary ethical issues that are currently relevant at your organization and that, if creatively addressed, would support physician and hospital staff in their roles?
3. What individuals at your organization or in your local area possess areas of ethics expertise, including the ability to put the theory and language of ethics into practice?
4. What measures for tracking ethical activity can be instituted at your organization this year and what resources are needed to gather, analyze, and educate key constituents based on this data?

NOTE

1. Other committee activities included: case consultation (19.9 percent), retrospective review of cases (14.9 percent), formulation and evaluation of policy (23.4 percent), and "other" (6.1 percent).

WORKS CITED AND RESOURCES

ASBH. American Society for Bioethics and Humanities. 1998. *Core competencies for health care ethics consultation.*

Churchill, L. R., and D. Schenck. 2005. One cheer for bioethics: Engaging the moral experiences of patients and practitioners beyond the big decisions. *Cambridge Quarterly of Healthcare Ethics* 14:389–403.

McGee, G., A. L. Caplan, J. P. Spanogle, and D. A. Asch. 2001. A national study of ethics committees. *American Journal of Bioethics* 1 (4): 60–64.

Rest, J. R., and D. Narvaez, eds. 1994. *Moral development in the professions: Psychology and applied.* 22–25.

Siegler, M. 1986. Ethics committees: Decisions by bureaucracy. *Hastings Century Report*16 (3): 22–24.

ADDITIONAL RESOURCES

Agich, G. J. 2001. The question of method in ethics consultation. *The American Journal of Bioethics* 1 (4): 31–41.

American Medical Association. 2004–2005. *Code of medical ethics current opinions with annotations.*

Lo, B. 2005. *Resolving ethical dilemmas: A guide for clinicians.* 3rd ed. Lippincott Williams & Wilkins.

President's Council on Bioethics. http://bioethics.gov/

Purtilo, R. B., G. M. Jensen, and B. Royeen. 2005. *Educating for moral action: A sourcebook in health and rehabilitation ethics.* F. A. Davis Company. Written for physical therapy and occupational therapy administrators, curriculum coordinators, and educators.

University of Washington School of Medicine. Ethics in medicine. http://depts.washington.edu/bioethx/toc.html.

11

Hospital Ethics Committees and Research with Human Beings

Timothy F. Murphy

KEY POINTS

1. To identify mechanisms of oversight for research involving human beings.
2. To identify the distinction between clinical innovation and formal research.
3. To identify some ways in which hospital ethics committees may involve themselves in innovative clinical therapy.

In the 1960s, the University of Washington established committees to evaluate candidates for a novel lifesaving technology that was rare at the time: hemodialysis (Jonsen 1992). The committees set standards to guide decisions about who got treatment and who did not. Critics of the process argued that the standards incorporated unfounded judgments about the value of some people's lives, which was especially problematic because the decisions literally meant the difference between life and death (Beam 2004; Pence 1980). As an antidote to these kinds of standards, some commentators wondered whether it would be better to introduce an element of chance into decisions about treatment (Childress 1979). At the very least, this approach would help avoid biases about whose lives were valuable and whose were not. As sometimes happens in the history of medicine, the ethical debate about these standards was not definitively resolved, with all parties coming to a satisfactory agreement that would stand the test of time. Instead, the debate was bypassed and rendered moot when the federal government stepped in during the 1970s and provided extensive contributions for payment of dialysis treatment (Rettig and Levinsky 1991). This approach resolved all difficult questions in deciding who would get dialysis on the basis of age, marital status, use of alcohol, and so on. After the government took this step, "God committees" that made decisions about dialysis simply went out of business, though the coverage provided by the federal government remained a matter of debate.

Despite their limited focus, these kinds of committees are in many ways a direct ancestor of today's hospital ethics committees (HECs). In the absence of identifiable standards for the allocation of scarce, life-saving technologies, physicians and institutions looked for counsel from experts in philosophy, theology, and the law. Some historians point to this outreach as the beginning of bioethics in its modern form (Jonsen 1998). Controversies about difficult medical decisions—including, for example, the feeding and hydration of newborns with severe disabilities as well as end-of-life care for adults—also drove professional interest in having some organized group available, to which health professionals could turn for guidance (Duff and Campbell 1973, 890–94). This need provided the conceptual space for HECs, and versions of these committees sprang up around the country. Since the 1990s, the Joint Commission on the Accreditation of Healthcare Organizations (JCAHO) requires that all medical institutions under its purview have in place a mechanism for the resolution of ethical conflicts, and most institutions turned to HECs as a way to do that.

During the same time when hospital committees were wrestling with hard questions of allocating life-saving technologies, a series of national scandals exposed the willful—or at least indifferent—exposure of human beings to harm in research. From the 1930s to the early 1970s, the Public Health Service, for example, conducted a natural history study of syphilis on poor African American men, in order to study the way the disease progressed, not to help the men themselves. The legacy of the Tuskegee syphilis studies—as these are known, for better or worse—interferes with good relationships between scientific researchers and African Americans to this day (Jones 1993). To cite one more example of reckless research, the Willowbrook studies—carried out under the direction of Saul Krimsky—involved the intentional feeding of hepatitis virus to institutionalized children with profound disabilities (Rothman and Rothman 2005). In response to these research scandals, in the late 1970s, the National Commission for the Protection of Human Subjects of Biomedical and Behavioral Research noted that healthcare researchers often made decisions about the design and conduct of research in the absence of any identifiable ethical standards, and the commission issued a number of reports in the 1970s to fill these voids.[1]

By now, of course, oversight committees are an established feature of the healthcare landscape, and it is the distinction between "clinical care" and "research" that frames the division of labor between committees. In general, HECs typically focus their skills and talents on difficult clinical decisions, institutional policies, and education rather than research. HECs came into existence in order to meet the internal needs of their individual institutions. By contrast, the recommendations that came out of the National Commission—including the influential Belmont Report—focus on ethical issues in research involving human beings, some of which is also the study of clinical care. The report called for the creation of local oversight bodies—Institutional Review Boards (IRBs)—in order to identify and deter objectionable research, and the federal government did go on to adopt regulations that apply to a great deal of research involving human subjects. As a result of this history, IRBs have the lion's share of responsibility for the oversight of research involving human beings. IRBs came into existence to satisfy federal sponsors of research that human beings were not inappropriately subjected to harm, either as individuals or as groups.

As things currently stand, HECs have no formal role to play when it comes to the review or approval of research properly speaking. That task belongs to IRBs, which have specific responsibilities in regard to informed consent, protection of confidentiality, and monitoring for safety. Even so, this division of labor leaves open some room for play. Existing oversight standards in research leave a good deal of discretion to clinicians in regard to innovative—even radically new—treatments for individual patients. In other words, IRBs do not have authority for prior review and approval over some treatments and innovations that are entirely new or new to an institution. These innovations may come to the attention of HECs for the reason that the clinicians involved wish to seek some counsel before going ahead with them. In these limited circumstances, HECs may have a role to play when it comes to the development or implementation of novel medical treatment.

OVERSEEING RESEARCH INVOLVING HUMAN BEINGS

In the United States, primary responsibility for oversight of research with human beings falls to IRBs, though in some cases, higher levels of review are required (for example, in research involving significant risks to healthy children) (Kopelman and Murphy 2004, 1–7). IRB responsibility extends to all research involving human subjects that is sponsored through federal funds that is conducted by institutions that have agreed to abide by these standards, to all privately funded research that involves bringing drugs and medical devices to market, and to research involving certain regulated substances such as ra-dioactive materials.[2] Even as broad as this umbrella of responsibility is, there remain some studies that do not require prior review and approval by an IRB. For example, some studies of educational prac-tices and certain kinds of anonymous social science surveys do not require prior review and approval by an IRB. Neither does the study of public behavior—for example, study of campaign appearances by politicians or the behavior of people in public venues—require prior review or approval. In the language of federal regulations, this kind of study is exempt from review by IRBs. Still, some institutions do have policies in place to ensure that their researchers do not exceed the boundaries of permissible research of this kind. They may re-quire, for example, academics engaged in this kind of study to de-scribe the study in detail, so that the institution can certify that it is exempt from IRB review.

While the scope of the regulations is broad, some study that is car-ried out for "in-house" purposes does not trigger the requirements for prior review and approval mentioned above. For example, a food company may wish to study the value of its line of diet foods. This study could involve following people for a period of time as they use these foods to determine how effective they are. Since the study does not use federal funds, use restricted substances, or otherwise trigger federal regulations, it remains beyond the domain of federal over-sight. Other studies—involving human beings or identifiable infor-mation about them—do not trigger the requirement of IRB review. As another example, if an institution wishes to study how many people acquire a viral or bacterial infection during their hospital stay, they may track all relevant medical records to do so, as frequently as they wish, without the knowledge or consent of the patients and without asking an IRB for prior review and approval. Their goal is not, strictly speaking, to make a contribution to generalizable knowledge, but to prevent these infections as far as possible through various interventions. By contrast, if an academic researcher at the hospital wanted to conduct the same study in the same hospital, IRB review would be required, if the reason for the study was to report findings to the public as a new contribution to professional knowledge. In short, federal regulations direct that IRBs review and approval certain kinds of research, but other domains of study are unregulated. Because some of this study could pose risks to the people involved, some commentators have argued for a more expansive standard, and in 2001, the National Bioethics Advisory Commission (NBAC) made exactly this recommendation.

At the same time, federal regulations go beyond defining what research must be reviewed and what is exempt. They also identify certain standards of membership and identify core functions for IRBs. In general, the membership of an IRB should have adequate scientific expertise and institutional knowledge to enable it to make reasonable evaluations about proposed research. If an IRB does not have the expertise to evaluate a particular research proposal, it may ask for help and advice from nonmembers, but ordinarily IRB membership should be equal to the task of evaluating the kinds of proposals it typically reviews. While there is no specific requirement, for example, that an IRB have a minimum number of physicians, it would only make sense to have multiple physicians involved in an IRB that oversaw a great deal of clinical experimentation. The IRB should also work to ensure representation of both male and female members and should have a member who is not otherwise affiliated with the sponsor institution. Other membership conditions may also apply. For example, if an IRB routinely evaluates research proposals involving the health and well-being of prisoners, federal regulations direct that an IRB should include someone knowledgeable about prisons and their populations.

IRBs are charged to evaluate research proposals with an eye toward protecting the rights and welfare of the men, women, and children involved. In particular, IRBs work to evaluate the ways in which subjects are recruited to the study and other aspects of the informed consent process that advises potential subjects about the risks and benefits of the research. IRBs also evaluate research proposals so that potential participants are advised of alternatives to participating in the research, their rights to withdraw from the research, and the identity of the people conducting the research. The IRB is also charged to ensure documentation of consent to participation in research, in a way that is proportionate to the risks of the study. An IRB may request modifications to a research proposal before granting approval to the study, and these modifications can extend to any matter the IRB believes will work to protect the rights and welfare of the subjects in the areas just mentioned.

IRBs are also charged to conduct reviews of all research they approve, at least once a year, but more frequently if the research involves, for example, medical risks that require close monitoring. (Researchers sometimes establish Data and Safety Monitoring Boards to do exactly this, and these boards evaluate the research at key points.) The IRB must also consider additional points of evaluation when it comes to the study of pregnant women, children, and wards of the state. Approval of any study does not mean that the study cannot be stopped. Just as the IRB has the responsibility to review and approve research before it begins, the IRB also may also suspend the research if, for example, it finds that the researchers have failed to abide by the terms of the study or that the expected risk-benefit calculation changes materially, to the detriment of the participants. It should also be noted that most IRBs are staffed by volunteers representing their own universities or medical centers. There is nothing in the federal regulations that requires volunteer IRBs, however, and a number of for-profit IRBs operate throughout the country (Emanuel 2006).

While the current system of IRB review has been in place for decades, it has its critics. Various academic commentators and federal commissions alike have studied the system and proposed a variety of changes. For example, commentators like Robert Levine have long argued that researchers should take more responsibility for the oversight of very low-risk research, in order to free up IRB time for the evaluation of more complex and risky research (Levine 1988). Other criticisms are even more far-reaching. In 2001, the NBAC proposed a series of significant changes in the current system of research oversight. For example, the commission recommended that the oversight system extend to all research that involves human beings in the United States, as previously mentioned, but it also recommended, for example, an accreditation mechanism for IRBs as well as standards for identifying and managing conflicts of interest, among other things. The commission also recommended unifying the federal oversight of research and stratifying research by degrees of risk in order to offer greater scrutiny to research that poses potentially higher degrees of risk (NBAC 2001). It is unclear what political traction any of these recommendations have behind them, and in fact, some efforts at change have already stalled. Even so, some changes in oversight standards may yet happen at some point in the future.

HOSPITAL ETHICS COMMITTEES, RESEARCH, AND CLINICAL INNOVATION

Insofar as research triggers the application of federal regulations or institutional policies, the responsibility to review and approve research involving human beings falls squarely on the shoulders of IRBs, not HECs. It is not the job of the HEC to review research protocols involving hospital patients, clinic patients, or anyone else. There is already a system in place to evaluate research proposals, from both scientific and ethical perspectives. In general, any projects that involve research—as defined by federal regulations and institutional policy—should be referred to IRBs.

Having said this, the division of labor between IRBs and HECs—roughly, research versus clinical care—does not mean that HECs never have a role to play in the emergence of new knowledge. One role that may occasionally fall to HECs emerges from the "play" left in federal regulations in regard to innovative clinical care.

The 1979 Belmont Report distinguished "research" from "clinical innovation" in order to differentiate investigation that should receive prior review from an oversight committee from medical care that should be exempted from that kind of review. According to this distinction, research is that work done to make a contribution to "generalizable knowledge." Ordinarily, this contribution is made through publications in scientific and academic journals or through formal communication with the professional community. By contrast, clinical innovations are those techniques and strategies a physician uses to take care of a specific individual patient, with perhaps no thought at all being given to communicating the outcome to the professional community. For example, a clinician may notice that all his diabetic patients share an unusual trait of the disease, something that has not been described in the scientific literature on diabetes. In order to learn whether that trait is part of the pathology of diabetes—or simply a coincidence in these patients—the physician may want to study a large number of people with diabetes, including the original patients. This investigation has the hallmarks of research properly speaking: it is designed and intended to answer a question of medical management that would be of interest to all physicians treating patients with diabetes, and the findings—if meaningful—would very likely be communicated to the medical community through professional journals.

By contrast, a physician might notice that the recommended dosages of a drug for patients with a certain disorder are either too high or too low for one of the patients in his or her practice. The physician might then vary the dosage in order to find a level that is effective for that particular patient. The issue at hand is what dosage is best for this particular patient. A physician might also wish to use a drug originally approved for one disorder for the treatment of another disorder altogether (this is known as "off-label" use), if he or she has good scientific reasons for doing so. Another example of clinical innovation might involve, for example, the use of a novel surgical technique with a patient with atypical liver anatomy. As these examples show, because of the vast number of ways in which people and treatments vary, clinicians will be called on throughout their practice to tailor unique, even innovative treatments—pharmaceutical and surgical—to individual patients. It is unreasonable to expect that they should seek prior review and approval for all novel choices they will make when treating patients.

In order to protect this domain of clinical judgment from unreasonable intrusion, the Belmont Report gives fairly wide berth to clinicians for individualized treatment. The report notes that "when a clinician departs in a significant way from standard or accepted practice, the innovation does not, in and of itself, constitute research. The fact that a procedure is 'experimental' in the sense of new, untested, or different, does not automatically place it in the category of research." The upshot of this conclusion is clear: not all novel medical interventions should be considered research properly speaking, and physicians may undertake even radically new innovations in the clinical care of individual patients so long as their goal is just that: taking care of individual patients.

This clinical freedom does not mean, however, that all physicians want to or should act completely independently and without counsel when initiating novel treatments. As a way of getting some measure of input regarding their innovative medical care, some clinicians want to turn to others for advice. It is in precisely this way that pioneers of medical therapy may interact with HECs. What clinicians may seek from HECs is not approval for research properly speaking but procedural advice about the best ways to protect patients undergoing planned innovative treatments. So long as the intended goal of the consultation is to offer advice regarding the care of an individual patient, physicians are free to consult HECs, and HECs are free to offer advice as they are equipped to do so. This advice might extend from the kind of informed consent process that should be used to the procedural safeguards that should be put in place to monitor the effect of the novel treatment.

Along these same lines, some commentators have proposed "innovative therapy committees" as forums in which clinicians can seek information useful to them prior to going forward with novel treatments. These committees would not be HECs properly speaking, but their function would be like the advisory role described above. The exact nature and role of innovative therapy committees is not well settled as a matter of professional consensus. Some commentators see them as intermediary committees, useful to clinicians in ways that IRB evaluation may not be (Reitsma and Moreno in press). Other commentators believe that IRBs should be involved in any ventures that involve novel treatments carried out with more than one patient. While the long-term fate of innovative therapy committees is unclear, it is worth saying that many clinicians may be uncertain about the boundaries between permitted clinical innovation and formal research properly speaking, or they may interpret the documents and language that establishes these domains in a number of ways. For example, surgeons might be unclear about what constitutes a routine variation on an established surgical technique and what constitutes major departure from established technique. In some professions, too, there is considerable background impetus to work toward innovation. Under such circumstances, it is not surprising that some physicians want to find a middle ground between independent judgment and the prior review required by IRBs, by looking to committees of peers for help. Some HECs already offer advice about the introduction of novel techniques and programs, but—in general—they should be reluctant to assume routine responsibility for the oversight of innovative therapy within any medical discipline just as they should avoid any function that duplicates—and therefore intrudes on—the work of IRBs.

It should also be noted that some healthcare professionals may turn to HECs when they wish to implement a program of medical care that is not novel per se. The medical treatment may be in use elsewhere at other hospitals or clinics, for example, but the treatment may be new to an institution and complex enough to warrant some scrutiny before making it available. For example, clinicians might bring a proposal regarding organ donation following cardiac death before HECs. Beyond soliciting advice about how to integrate the novel medical care within an institution, physicians may also turn to HECs to solicit participation in their medical programs. One university hospital has reported that its HEC participated in the introduction of its living liver donor program and went on to assume a direct role in that program (Anderson-Shaw et al. 2005). The staff of the transplant program first evaluates potential donors for their medical and psychological suitability to donate a portion of their liver to a family member or friend. When cleared in those ways to donate, a member of the HEC conducts an independent interview with the potential donor to try to detect whether the donor really wants to go forward with the surgery and whether there are any undue influences or any elements of coercion in the donor's decision. The HEC member reports any concerns of this kind or any apparent deficits in the donor's understanding of the procedure back to the transplant team, as well as any concerns the donor has that have not been addressed to that point.

In addition to the roles that HECs sometimes assume in offering consultation regarding novel clinical care or novel treatment programs, HECs may have yet one more role to play when it comes to the oversight of research involving human beings. As noted above, the Belmont Report identified a domain of clinical care in which clinicians are free to make decisions regarding the care of individual patients. But the authors of the report were also aware of the need for evaluating those innovations and so went on to say that "radically new procedures of this description should, however, be made the object of formal research at an early stage, in order to determine whether they are safe and effective. Thus, it is the responsibility of medical practice committees, for example, to insist that a major innovation be incorporated into a formal research project." In other words, clinical innovations should be subjected to formal research early on, to assess their value generally. It would be unfortunate if one clinician's innovation came into widespread use—through word of mouth or case study reports—without good evidence that the treatment was of general benefit compared to its risks, which—unfortunately—is exactly what sometimes happens, as in the case of a widely used surgery later shown to have very limited benefit (Moseley et al. 2002). The Belmont Report charged medical practice committees to take the lead in ensuring that innovations are formally studied as soon as practical, but HECs may sometimes be aware of innovative medical procedures and be in a position to make a recommendation that clinicians move toward formal study of a novel intervention as well.

CONCLUSION

In the United States, IRBs are and will remain the central bodies having the responsibility to evaluate and monitor research involving human beings. Their specific responsibilities have not changed substantially since the system of IRB oversight was first put in place in the 1970s, but because of continuing discussions about the exact nature of their work, it would not be surprising if some changes are eventually adopted. Even if some changes do occur, the broad outlines of IRB responsibilities are likely to remain intact for the foreseeable future: their primary responsibility will be to protect the rights and welfare of human beings under study in research. To ensure that IRBs are equal to that task, some education is typically required for membership, and this education usually consists of study of the relevant sections of the *Code of Federal Regulations*, the Belmont Report, or even short research ethics courses dealing with such issues as examples of abuse, standards of informed consent, vulnerable populations, and community consultation. Armed with a common vocabulary, standards, and purpose, IRBs review research proposals in order to ensure that people understand what is being asked of them in research, that risks are fully identified and balanced carefully against potential benefits, that access and equity in subject recruitment are protected, and that research is monitored in proportion to its potential risks. The federal Office for Human Research Protections offers considerable guidance to IRBs in these matters.[3] Even though this guidance does not always have the force of regulation, it still functions as a statement of best practices when it comes to research ethics.

All in all, the United States has a formidable infrastructure capable of identifying and deterring objectionable research, even if questions remain about how well it functions at every level. (Some commentators worry, for example, about variability among individual IRBs and the burden multiple IRB review places on research conducted at multiple sites around the country.) By contrast, most HECs across the country do not share a common charge. Not even the JCAHO requirement that institutions have a mechanism to resolve ethical conflicts requires that these institutions have HECs properly speaking. Institutions might meet this requirement, for example, simply by offering an ethics consultation service, staffed by various people with various backgrounds. Neither do HECs share set of common regulations or policies to help guide their activities and decision making, and there can be no expectation that members of HECs across the country share any kind of common educational experience to prepare them for their committee service. Some members of HECs will have experience serving on an IRB and the education that goes with that, but in some institutions, there may be no overlap at all in membership between HECs and IRBs.

This is to say that—all things considered—HECs are widely variable in membership, educational preparation, and core activities. In the absence of national standards defining their work, there is a wide spectrum in what HECs actually do and how they accomplish their work. To be sure, some HECs are more ambitious than others and carry out extensive educational activities, work continuously on refining institutional policies, and provide more or less immediate consultation regarding clinical care. By contrast, other HECs are far less developed and involved with their institutions; they function with far fewer resources and—as a result—achievements. Because of this wide variation, HECs can look very different from one another in their overall vitality and role in an institution.

As a matter of federal regulations and institutional policies, HECs do not play any formal role in the oversight of research involving human beings. Any HEC that approved a research project involving human beings on its own would almost certainly violate federal regulations or institutional policies. HECs should refer to IRBs any requests for evaluation of proposed research involving human participants. They already have enough to do anyway. HECs trace their roots to the need for an institutional forum for the discussion of difficult clinical decisions, useful educational programs, and needed institutional policies. In an environment that changes quickly—because of technological innovation, modifications to the law, and social debate—these concerns will remain the core activities of HECs for the foreseeable future.

Even so, HECs can play a role in the emergence of new knowledge and medical practices, as happens when clinicians solicit advice about proposed medical procedures that are novel in their own right or new to an institution. Discussing these matters does not constitute an oversight role in research properly speaking, and there is nothing inherently problematic about HECs offering advice as it pertains to, for example, informed consent for a novel endocrine surgery. In responding to requests for this kind of advice, any HEC should of course make sure that its expertise is equal to the complexities of the intervention in question. HECs can decline to become involved in these kinds of discussion if they believe the matters lay beyond their expertise or compromise other work they do. As they do this kind of consultation, if HECs discover clinical activities that amount to research properly speaking, but that have not received prior review and approval, they should immediately counsel the professionals involved to contact the appropriate oversight body without delay. HECs should also keep in mind that they may have a role to play in urging clinicians who do use novel therapies to subject them to formal evaluation at the earliest possible opportunity, in keeping with the Belmont Report's advisory on the subject.

As they engage in these various activities, HECs should also keep in mind that they may sometimes open themselves up to the appearance of conflicts of interest: in making recommendations on a given medical treatment or program, is an HEC working to advance the interests of the institution or to protect the patients involved? Enthusiasm for institutional advance may—just may—cloud advice about what standards and practices best protect patients facing novel or complex treatment. No less than other advisory bodies, HECs should always work to avoid actual and apparent conflicts of interest to the extent possible, and they can do this by committing themselves in an undivided way to the welfare of patients above all else.

FOR FURTHER REFLECTION

1. Dr. Sandra Edwards approaches her HEC and asks its advice about implementing a pediatric bariatric surgery program. She is especially interested in surgery that permanently reduces the

size of the stomach. The use of this surgery in children is not well studied for its long-term effects, but several medical centers around the country now use it, and Dr. Edwards wants to know whether she should consider the procedure experimental.

2. Dr. Jason Luo has noticed that four of his patients are responding well to a drug regimen that is not described anywhere in the professional literature. He has given these patients drugs approved by the Food and Drug Administration for other purposes. He approaches his HEC and asks whether they would like to receive reports on the outcome as he treats these patients with this regimen.

3. As a general question, is there any reason to think that HECs should assume greater responsibilities for the clinical experimentation that goes on in their institutions? What are some reasons that this might be a good idea? Are there any reasons this would not be a good idea?

NOTES

1. See http://www.bioethics.gov/reports/past_commissions/index.html.

2. The relevant sections describing the standards for oversight of research are at 45 *Code of Federal Regulations* 46 and 21 *Code of Federal Regulations* 50.

3. See www.hhs.gov/ohrp/.

WORKS CITED

Anderson-Shaw, L., M. L. Schmidt, J. Elkins, et al. 2005. Evolution of a living donor liver transplantation advocacy program. *Journal of Clinical Ethics* 16 (1): 46–57.

Beam, T. E. 2004. Medical ethics on the battlefield: The crucible of military medical ethics. *Military Medical Ethics* 1:369–402.

Childress, J. F. 1979. Who shall live when not all can live? *Soundings* 62:258–69.

Department of Health, Education, and Welfare. *The Belmont Report.* 1979. http://poynter.indiana.edu/sas/res/belmont.html.

Duff, R. S.; and A. G. M. Campbell. 1973. Moral and ethical dilemmas in the special care nursery. *New England Journal of Medicine* 289:890–94.

Emanuel, E. J. 2006. Should society allow research ethics boards to be run as for-profit enterprises? *PLoS Biology* 4:7, pe309.

Jones, J. 1993. *Bad blood: The Tuskegee syphilis experiment.* 2nd ed. New York: Free Press.

Jonsen, A. R. 1992. *The new medicine and the old ethics.* Cambridge: Harvard University Press.

————. 1998. *The birth of bioethics.* Oxford: Oxford University Press.

Kopelman, L. M., and T. F. Murphy. 2004. Ethical concerns about federal approval of risky pediatric studies. *Pediatrics* 113 (6): 1–7.

Levine, R. J. 1988. *Ethics and regulation of clinical research.* 2nd ed. New Haven, CT: Yale University Press.

Moseley, J. B., K. O'Malley, N. J. Petersen, et al. 2002. A controlled trial of arthroscopic surgery for osteoarthritis of the knee. *New England Journal of Medicine* 347 (2): 81–88.

NBAC. National Bioethics Advisory Commission. 2001. *Ethical and policy issues in research involving human participants.* Washington, DC: National Bioethics Advisory Commission. Available at http://www.georgetown.edu/research/nrcbl/nbac/pubs .html.

Pence, G. E. 1980. *Classic cases in medical ethics.* New York: McGraw-Hill.

Reitsma, A. M., and J. D. Moreno, eds. 2006. *Ethical guidelines for innovative surgery.* Hagerstown, MD: University Publishing Group.

Rettig, R. A., and N. G. Levinsky, eds. 1991. *Kidney failure and the federal government.* Washington, DC: Institute of Medicine Press.

Rothman, D. J., and S. M. Rothman. 2005. *The Willowbrook wars: Bringing the mentally disabled into the community.* Somerset, NJ: Aldine Transaction.

12

Distributive Justice in Hospital Healthcare

Michael Boylan and Richard E. Grant

KEY POINTS

1. Core concerns include policy, education, and clinical case consultation in light of a community worldview that includes distributive justice.
2. Hospital ethics committees (HECs) should situate their perspectives into a global context that will extend beyond their own individual hospital.
3. HECs should seek to ration health care as much as possible upon cooperative rather than competitive criteria.

Today the United States is faced with a "good news and bad news" scenario. On the one hand, we have more resources than we have ever had before, and a goodly portion is being directed toward health care. On the other hand, our medical advances are so significant that we have moved into a situation in which there are healthcare options that are too expensive to provide to all. The core concerns of HECs are to advise on policy, education, and clinical case consultation. This chapter contends that in order to perform these tasks authentically, the concerns of the environment in which the hospital operates and the context of justice are critical. These concerns leave us to ascertain how best to allocate resources among patients and institutions. In order to provide a reasonable scheme for allocation, we turn, then, to principles of distributive justice.

A decided focus on principled reflection is paramount. That is, HECs should consider issues of resource allocation specifically according to general principles and not simply in a pragmatic, ad hoc fashion. This is because the latter devolves into a political spoils system in which the most adept claimants can garner the most resources. Now, some might claim, "What's the matter with that? Isn't that just democracy?" In reply, the authors would charge that blatant manipulation of power is best described as "kraterism." The term comes from the classical Greek term *kratein* meaning "to prevail by getting the upper hand through the use of power." A kraterist is the sort of person embodied by two characters from the dialogues *Republic* and *Gorgias*, by the ancient Greek philosopher, Plato (1903). Therein, Plato develops arguments for and against kraterism through the guises of Thrasymachus and Callicles. Specifically, these individuals hold that justice is the rule of the strongest—a position found wanting by Plato's protagonist, Socrates. In our modern world, kraterism is readily displayed under the rule of dictators. In fact, "Justice is the rule of the strongest" may be well characterized as the mantra of dictators. The authors of this chapter believe that the worldview of these individuals is a form of social Darwinism—which itself is problematic.

On the one hand, the kraterist worldview has the advantage that it is pure and unmixed. It is all about the satisfaction of egoism. Kraterists typically view the mythical state of the world as very hostile and believe that only the strong survive. Since they don't want to be among those who fail, they are willing to do what it takes to succeed. They want to get paid big money to take big risks. Success is the only justification within kraterism, and one doesn't know if one has made it until the game's over. On the other hand, in order to protect their position, kraterists often create a phony situation of entrapment. It is the typical response of the kraterist. When confronted with their actions, they try to outflank their opponent instead of changing their behavior.

Now it is clear that kraterism greatly resembles capitalism ("to each according to his valued work"). The critical term in the capitalist allocation formula is "valued." Since most agents value what they do (or want to do) above all else, this allocation scheme requires some independent setting of value. This is usually done by power manipulators (advertisers and politicians). They try to influence popular perceptions of social value so that these power brokers win. In this way, capitalism is dependent upon kraterism for its operation. Both must be seen together as representing competitive theories of distributive justice. Advocates of this position think *all* allocation is competitive, whether in health care or other institutions. The authors of this chapter believe such a position to be false, missing the cooperative character constitutive of health care as a field. "Allocation" is not reducible to competition. Various entities can request money from a common source while recognizing that some claims will (and ought to) trump others. The recognition and acceptance of this is the beginning of the other large class of distribution: cooperative theories.

The best-known cooperative theories are economic socialism and egalitarianism (Boylan 2004). The mission of medicine under ancient and contemporary sources is not competitive, but cooperative.[1] The principles of beneficence, nonmaleficence, fostering autonomy, and justice are grounded on cooperative premises (Beauchamp and Childress 2001; Boylan 2000). Since medicine's mission is cooperative, the position taken in this chapter is that kraterism and capitalism are not the appropriate foundational sources for medical resource allocation. Instead, some cooperative formula must be fashioned. This formula must be set out in the context of today's medical community. While some of the issues discussed in this chapter are beyond the policy prerogative of the HECs, we believe that committee members are better served by understanding the larger context of their discussions and deliberations so that they might more coherently and authentically make decisions affecting the hospitals they serve.

HOSPITALS TODAY

In order to arrive at a cooperative theory of resource allocation that is just, we must assess the current mission of the most prevalent hospital types operating in the United States. Generically, each hospital has certain basic needs: (a) personnel: physicians, nurses, support staff; (b) basic accommodations: rooms, beds, food, and an unpolluted interior atmosphere; (c) medicines, both ordinary and extraordinary; (d) diagnostic and treatment devices; (e) an operating room and emergency department (ED); (f) other specialized equipment and personnel according to various specialized needs; and (g) a billing and collections department. Beyond these basic requirements some hospitals have specialized needs based upon their unique missions. To simplify our discussion, we group them by the following types: teaching, community, public and VA hospitals.

Teaching hospitals have three missions: to (a) care for the sick, (b) train new physicians, and (c) extend human knowledge through laboratory and clinical research. These hospitals are very expensive to operate since the sorts of resources they require include increased facilities for students, more basic medical supplies (since this situation creates structural inefficiencies), state-of-the-art diagnostic and treatment equipment to train the physicians, and all the supplies necessary for keeping a lab going.

Community hospitals are often private hospitals that serve affluent populations that generally possess health insurance. Most of the resource needs reduce to the generic model with the exception that sometimes these hospitals will specialize in one area of medicine (such as cardiology) and therefore require specialized facilities to support this specific focus.

Public hospitals, both urban and rural, are funded by government and other sources and provide the majority of care for the poor and uninsured. Given the financial status of these patients, many use the emergency department of these hospitals for primary care. Because of the necessity of providing primary care to their patient population, these hospitals often emphasize basic medical supplies over more extraordinary medical equipment because more people can be treated under that allocation strategy. These hospitals may also have to overinvest in the billing and collections side of the house in order to stay in business. Additional personnel requirements may include social workers who can connect families to government and private programs that can also provide help.

Veterans Administration (VA) hospitals have as their special mission the care of military personnel and their families—with emphasis on care of injuries and disabilites sustained during service. Particular resource needs include more equipment and personnel in rehabilitation and psychiatric services. There are also overlapping profiles of the inner-city and rural hospitals, since many of our veterans in the era of the all-volunteer army are from the lowest two quintiles of income (as per the GINI Index, see Alker 1965).

FOR-PROFIT AND NOT-FOR-PROFIT HOSPITALS

The division of hospital types focuses primarily on both mission and populations served. However, with the focus of this chapter on resource allocation, it is also worth looking at hospitals according to financial structure, specifically whether a hospital is "for profit" or "not for profit." Though all public and all VA hospitals are not for profit, community and teaching hospitals may be private for profit, private not for profit, or public not for profit.

For-profit hospitals are designed to provide high-end care that also succeeds at making money for corporations and even shareholders. They are often run by multistate corporations or a hospital management company. For-profit hospitals frequently expand their operations by absorbing community hospitals and developing a new charter for operations. Large hospital centers prefer to manage themselves unless the hospital is facing imminent demise or extreme economic distress. Health maintenance organizations and management companies have had difficulty in the recent decade because large physicians' groups have rebelled against their punitive financial models. Alternatively, physicians have developed their own large health maintenance organizations to manage their physician-owned hospitals.

When a hospital becomes a for-profit entity, it must fight the tendency to evolve into the kraterism extreme regardless of its original business model or mission statement. An example of this might be the Columbia/HCA Corporation case from the mid-1990s. Columbia/HCA was the largest for-profit healthcare corporation in America with as many as 340 hospitals in its company. A government probe of Columbia/HCA found systematic and criminal fraud in Medicare billings. This example alone serves as a reminder of the importance of monitoring the day-to-day operations and strategic planning at and by all administrative levels (including HECs) in for-profit hospitals in order to avoid these tendencies that originate from the imperative to focus on the bottom line even if companies are not publicly traded. These for-profit hospital systems provide health-care services for their patients and bill Medicaid and Medicare and commercial insurance companies to underwrite their economic activities.

Because of the dual mission of medicine and business, the HECs at for-profit hospitals should weigh the issue of distributive justice in light of the *medical* mission of the hospital: to heal the sick and the injured through the expression of sympathetic goodwill. This sympathetic goodwill can often work against the profit model since it would dictate caring without asking how or whether the patient can pay the bill. The patient's care comes first. This outcome needs constant monitoring—especially at for-profit hospitals.

Obviously, when one puts the patient's care first, then profits can decrease and an often unstated part of the for-profit hospital mission statement, which dictates securing a working profit, will be unfulfilled. Thus, the tendency is toward profits coming first, and this leads to kraterism. If we are correct about this tendency, then it is up to HECs to monitor operations and patient care to make sure that the hospital continues to live up to its medical mission.

Not-for-profit hospitals contrast directly with the for-profit model. A clear difference in institutional worldview perspective can be found if we focus on public (or county) hospital systems where the economic support is underwritten by grants from nonprofit organizations and resources emanating from the federal or state government. Examples of funding foundation grants include the Joyce Foundation, the Robert Wood Johnson Foundation, the MacArthur Foundation, or the Ford Foundation. Often, foundations become the principal financial underwriter of public hospitals, thereby supplementing this system's limited federal funding. Examples of federal funding include monies obtained by public hospital systems through the Bureau of Health Resource Services under the U.S. Department of Health and Human Services (HHS). These entities, once considered expansive pockets of money, have been shrinking inexorably since the latter part of the Clinton era (1998–2000). HHS controls Medicaid and Medicare and the CMS Division, and as a department in the federal government, ultimate control is under the power of political appointees. Sometimes political appointees thwart traditional practice and policies (see Weisman 2005, A-1).[2] Thus, allocation decisions that operated on one set of assumptions under one administration can change in another. HECs need to stay abreast of these trends, working with ombudsmen to monitor the reactions of senior hospital administrators to these trends.

The country's rural hospitals are invariably public hospital systems and are funded by federal and local entities. For most public hospitals such as county hospital systems, the need for public funding becomes central to the mission of the hospital. Any county hospital system receiving federal funds must operate in accordance with an implied mandate corresponding to the mission of that class of hospital. Such hospitals must allow for the treatment of at least 3 to 4 percent of their patient population that is designated within the category of being "underserved." In addition, publicly funded hospitals with a public funding charter must treat all emergencies entering their premises. HECs should carefully monitor this outcome to ensure compliance.

Public and county hospital systems are considered "safety net hospitals."[3] The mission of most safety net hospitals is to provide comprehensive health care for underserved populations—serving in full capacity as an unabashed "public hospital." However, these hospitals are either closing or not keeping pace with population trends relating to their target population of economically disadvantaged individuals. On the aggregate level, a recent report by the Robert Wood Johnson Foundation covering the years 1996–2002 showed that public hospitals are down by 27 percent in poverty suburbs and 16 percent in urban areas of poverty (Andrulis and Duchon 2005). The number of for-profit hospitals that service primarily populations in wealthier demographic groups are about to surpass nonprofit hospitals for the first time. The report further concludes that high-poverty communities in the cities or in the suburbs are being underserved in medical care compared with more affluent populations. This finding suggests that our social medical safety net is rapidly disintegrating. These aggregate numbers can be better put into perspective by examining an extended example from the Chicago area.

Cook County in Illinois is charged with underwriting the mission of its county hospital system using taxpayers' money. Currently, Cook County Hospital provides the tax revenue dollars that underwrite 35 percent of the Cook County Hospital System budget, though this percentage is down from 50 percent in just the past few years (Stroger 2005). The remainder of the county safety net budget is derived from Medicare and Medicaid funding in addition to third-party insurance payers. Thus, non–tax dollar resources must now account for at least 65 percent of the Cook County Hospital System's budget by 2005 (Stroger 2005). Obviously, the apportionment from different payers suggests (as noted in the Robert Wood Johnson Report) that a great majority of the underserved population are not receiving proper medical care. Those among the underserved who are excluded from the current budget scheme are either dying prematurely or not receiving any care at all. The trend in most urban areas is to provide less money for the underinsured. Obviously, the underinsured have become very resourceful in identifying ways through the healthcare labyrinth. Several have attempted to solve their healthcare needs by seeking alternative services and alternative treatments.

Per the details in the Robert Wood Johnson Report, most public hospitals are burdened with a huge volume of patients who overwhelm existing emergency care services. Cook County's ED patients wait for hours in order to receive care because they are often unable to obtain or afford care through private physicians. The urban hospital emergency care area becomes the default primary care provider for the underinsured.[4]

During 2004 in Cook County, there were at least 227,000 emergency care visits. Provident Hospital in Chicago had 50,000 emergency care visits and 22,800 admissions (Provident Hospital website 2005). Typically, public hospitals or county hospital centers are characterized by emergency care areas that are overwhelmed by the sheer volume of uninsured patients. Frequently, the uninsured patient will seek care at a county hospital system to obtain free primary care or treatment of sexually transmitted diseases that may be embarrassing and have untoward social consequences. When patients wish to remain anonymous and have the sexually transmitted diseases resolved, they will often seek out the services of county public health centers or county hospital emergency rooms. Safety net county hospital emergency care treatment areas often receive patients with AIDS or AIDS-related diseases in addition to other sexually transmitted diseases, cancer, and illegal aliens seeking medical care.

Health provider manpower at Cook County Hospital is often supplied by residents (physicians still completing graduate medical education) working within the Cook County system. Local medical schools often contract with the county hospital system to provide medical education for their residents. Cook County has an open policy with respect to resident education suggesting that any bona fide teaching hospital can contact the administrators at the Cook County Hospital System and request that Cook County provide an educational site for resident medical training activities. Usually, the residents' salaries are paid for by the sponsoring institution.

Since the goal of public hospitals is to be interested in delivering the best care according to the generally accepted tenets of public health care, which involves assessing the community's needs and then identifying those resources that are available and matching the needs of the community, they must always adopt policy strategies that seek to obtain the greatest amount of impact per healthcare dollar. The public health emphasis for most public hospitals is to remain focused on preventive care, which turns out to be much more cost effective than tertiary care and prolonged hospitalization for acute, multiple system failures.

The public hospital system that services poverty populations must recognize the reality of their shrinking financial support. The above case example illustrates the mechanics of this. Further, HEC members must be aware of their individual situation within this milieu. This is because ethical decisions do not exist in a vacuum. The core concerns of policy, education, and clinical case consultation must be seen within these contexts.

UNDERSTANDING THE MILIEU

At the end of the last section, it was suggested that HEC members need to contextualize their duties to provide policy guidance, education, and clinical case consultation. This is because the manner in which they can and should execute their task is limited by these parameters, but the reflective considerations also occur within an expansive and complex milieu, some features of which will be discussed below.

CHRONIC ILLNESS—URBAN AND RURAL

One important feature was suggested at the end of the last section on the allocation of clinical resources with public health understandings in mind. The approach to hospital policies on chronic illness may depend upon this dynamic. As our ability to extend life has improved, there has been a direct rise in the incidence of chronic illnesses. However, it should be noted that at least 80 percent of chronic illnesses are preventable, such as hypercholesterolemia, hypertension, adult-onset diabetes mellitus, chronic obstructive pulmonary disease, asthma, and some neoplasms. If one evaluates the ten leading causes of death in the United States, which consume the majority of the available healthcare dollars, they account for a massive expenditure of money during hospitalization in the end stage of critical care precipitated by years of neglect or inadequate or inappropriate care (Lubtiz and Riley 1993; Scitovsky 1984, 1994; Barnato et al. 1999). Most public health advocates attempt to determine the means by which they might prevent patients from arriving at the point of neglect and chronicity of disease requiring acute hospital admissions to a critical care or intensive care unit. It is worth noting that many of those who are incarcerated throughout the United States prison systems receive better treatment during incarceration than economically disadvantaged persons who are not in prison. Prisoners are provided a comprehensive program of healthcare and measures for preventive health care, are instituted throughout the time in the prison system (Lindquist 1999).

MEDICAL LIABILITY, MALPRACTICE INSURANCE, AND TORT REFORM

Another issue looming in the future with respect to hospitals that HECs need to take into consideration with respect to clinical case consultation is the current malpractice climate. The cost of rising malpractice insurance is of concern to both hospitals and physicians. For example, in urban areas such as Philadelphia, the average cost of malpractice insurance for private practice orthopedists is approximately $250,000 per year. By contrast, the cost is approximately $197,000 per year for orthopedists who are members of a hospital staff and covered under the hospital's blanket insurance trust (American Hospital Association website). However, it stands to reason that, within a teaching institution paying at least $197,000 for faculty members teaching orthopedic residents, the relationship between the hospital administration and the department of orthopedic surgery changes considerably, as the administration will, of course, shift the emphasis from teaching and education of residents to faculty productivity, RVUs, and CPT codes. Certainly, the tort climate does affect the way medicine is practiced. It should be of utmost importance to HECs to evaluate grand rounds sessions and create (if they are not already in place) "ethics grand rounds" that discuss the hospital's position with respect to policy relating to difficult case types. The legal staff of the hospital should be brought in on this so that the entire hospital team works to prevent needless loss of resources on frivolous cases and provide proactive compensation in those cases with merit. Remember, most lawsuits can be contained (even in at-fault cases) when goodwill and quick response are invoked.

WORLD HEALTH

Of course, the medical milieu transcends the borders of our country. A recent article in *The Washington Post* documented that the World Health Organization (WHO) has identified millions of deaths that are preventable (Weisman 2005). Nearly 400 million people will die of heart disease, diabetes, and other chronic ailments within the next ten years but many of these deaths could be prevented by lifestyle changes and inexpensive medications. The financial burden from an increasing death toll from such noncommunicable diseases will present an enormous cost to emerging countries such as India and China. It is estimated that the cost to such evolving countries will be in the billions of dollars. The WHO has called attention to the increasing threat from noncommunicable diseases that account for three out of five deaths worldwide. They insist that these deaths can be prevented by healthful diets, forsaking tobacco use, exercise, and inexpensive medications.

Previously, such conditions were overshadowed by infectious diseases such as HIV/AIDS that cause far more deaths. The WHO estimated that 39 million deaths from chronic disease in the next ten years could be prevented, including 28 million of these deaths in developing countries such as India and China.

The point here for HECs is that within their hospital class, each hospital must see its mission in the context of the global mission of health care. This may mean creating ways of helping elsewhere. In the case of public and VA hospitals, this may be impossible because their own needs are overwhelming. But in the case of solvent teaching and community hospitals (and certainly for-profit hospitals that are making a profit), such obligations must be seen as action-guiding.

THE PROBLEM OF RATIONING

We might say that what has been discussed so far is the necessary background for the central issue of the chapter and HECs to consider.

In light of cooperative principles of just distribution, the hospital environment in which HECs operate, and the medical milieu present in the United States and beyond, the issue that all HECs must accept from the outset in their policy and education roles is that there will always be greater legitimate claims for health care than there are resources to provide such care. This is true the world over. The consequence of this is that clear allocation strategies must be in place. Most of these are out of the hands of individual hospitals (residing at the state and federal level). Because of this, the individual hospital's allocation strategy must be "reactionary." By reactionary, we mean that one must react to the social and political environment in fashioning rationing strategies for the individual hospital.

Now, the word "rationing" has a very bad ring to most individuals when talking about healthcare resource allocation. This is because of our cultural emphasis on individual choice and the nature of the individual rights claim. We contend that individual rights claims are only appropriate to goods that are related to action. That is, there is a (moral) hierarchy of claims to goods that may be ranked according to their proximity to action. Although elsewhere, the complete argument for basing everything upon the grounds of action is given in more detail (Boylan 2004), a taste of this argument for providing goods to all agents according to their proximity to the grounds of action is sketched in the endnotes.[5] For our immediate purposes, fundamental human rights claims can be schematically set out as follows:

The Table of Embeddedness[6]

I. Basic Goods
   A. Level One: food, clothing, shelter, protection from unwarranted bodily harm (including access to health care).
   B. Level Two: basic education (primary and secondary) and human freedom.
II. Secondary Goods
   A. Level One: Equal opportunity to pursue education (tertiary), employment, and life plan to self-fulfillment.
   B. Level Two: Obtaining goods equivalent to others in a socially similar situation (keeping up with the Joneses).
   C. Level Three: Obtaining goods in excess to others in a socially similar situation (exceeding the Joneses).

The purpose of keeping such a schematic table in mind as a member of an HEC is that it forms the basis of distributive justice and hence provides the theoretical grounding behind rationing. Rationing should be grounded upon the hierarchical claims for goods that all individuals can make. The most basic of these claims must always trump the less essential. This principle is similar to standard clinical triage, and, ethically, is more generally depicted by the Table of Embeddedness. More specifically, the issue of justice (viewed from the standpoint of society) with regard to health care is that if each person has a right to health care, then perhaps health care, itself, has its own table of embeddedness that is weighted not only on its relation to agency (since presumably all healthcare needs threaten agency) but according to how many people's needs can be met.

Because there is no justification based on either aggregation or on pleasure, as such, this is not a principle of utilitarianism that grounds rights claims on the basis of social utility—the greatest good for the greatest number. Rather, it is a policy assessment of how many valid rights claims can be met. Since all health claims threaten agency in some degree, one would like to satisfy as many as possible. In most hospitals, this is described as a triage formula. As this essay has suggested, the needs of various hospitals makes it impossible to impose a universal triage formula. This is because triage is based upon a needs-vs.-resources matrix. In the best possible situation, we would treat those in greatest need first and then work backward. But in situations in which there are far too few dollars to handle the mission of the hospital, then there needs to be a readjustment. The HEC should be at the forefront of such a readjustment.

In assessing the theory behind any readjustment, let us for simplicity say that medical claimants come in three classes: primary, intermediate, and acute care. Each class must claim an equal portion of the hospital's resources. This may mean that some individuals in each class might be denied care. This is because rationing is necessary: there is not enough money to support everyone. However, it is the conjecture of these authors that in most hospital types, most of the rationing will occur at the level of acute care.

Since all claimants at any level have an equal claim to health care, then it is the case that an arbitrary choice process must be instituted. This so-called lottery mechanism should be class blind. When we have one hundred claimants and only enough resources to service ninety, then ten will not receive adequate care for their needs. As a result, they may die. But if the random selection procedure is fair and transparent, then there is no legitimate blame, except against "bad luck," both through the illness or accident and through one's missing out on the healthcare lottery.

These are hard realities. No one wants to confront another person and say that there is no healthcare solution available because we don't have the resources (especially given that we are the richest nation on earth). We must be vigilant that the process is not skewed toward those with the ability to pay (the affluent), resulting in kraterism.

Instead, the ethics committees should recommend that cooperative theories of justice such as egalitarianism (equal treatment in each class of claimant) and socialism (traditional triage distribution according to need) be employed. This should be the overarching principle for all ethics committees:

> To each class of medical claimants (primary, intermediate, and acute) equally, and within each class according to need, subject to "ought implies can," in which case, a random distribution formula should be applied.

This is a bold statement about a controversial position because it takes people where they are and does not attempt to judge or punish them for behavior that may have put them there (see further Boylan 2004). We advocate this distribution formula as being the most fair.

CONCLUSION

It is difficult to create one template upon which all possibilities can be sorted. There are various sorts of hospitals. This essay has set out four classes of hospitals that can, in turn, be set into two groups. The second group (public hospitals and VA hospitals) are in an acute rationing mode. We suggest allocation directions for them. In the first group: teaching hospitals and community hospitals that are making money (as well as all for-profit hospitals); some of the needs of the larger community should be considered when these hospitals are able to meet their own needs. These hospitals should contribute to the resources of the larger national and international community, which are so short of resources that it is a clear injustice that people die because of lacking basic primary care. This is not just someone else's problem. The medical community must adopt a worldview of cooperation. This means that the hospital community should operate according to Martin Luther King Jr.'s dictum that "injustice anywhere is a threat to justice everywhere." We must all be an active part of the solution. The shared community worldview of each hospital should be the promotion of health, and the curing of illness and accident, to people first in their own domain, then to those in their vicinity, next to others in their country, and finally to the general human community.

FOR FURTHER REFLECTION

1. How can our HEC integrate theoretical concepts of distributive justice into our day-to-day operation?
2. How might our HEC integrate national and global considerations of justice into our policies, procedures, and institutional outreach?
3. Since it is a given that health care must be rationed, how can we create an ethical procedure that meets the hospital's mission and also the ethical sensibilities of HEC members?

NOTES

1. A sympathetic argument from a different standpoint is made by Hester on the subject of residency matching in two articles (2001, 2003).

2. There are an increasing number of these cases. For example, according to USA Today.com (May 6, 2004, accessed May 8, 2006), the FDA's politically appointed commissioners overruled the recommendations of their career scientists about the hazards of allowing the "morning after pill" to be sold "over the counter." In another case, the Bush administration officials overrode WHO recommendations for more condoms to fight AIDS in Uganda. Instead, political appointees wanted the extra money spent upon abstinence programs (this despite the recommendations of career public health officials, New York Times.com, August 30, 2005, accessed May 9, 2006).

3. Examples would include DC General, Washington, DC; Cook County Hospital, Chicago, Illinois; Charity Hospital, New Orleans, Louisiana; and Grady Hospital, Atlanta, Georgia.

4. An example would be Provident Hospital in south side Chicago, Illinois, which has become the second-busiest emergency care area in the entire Chicago, Illinois area (Provident Hospital website 2005).

5. Boylan's argument for this is (2004, ch. 3):

1. Before all else, all people desire to act—Fact
2. Whatever all people desire before anything else is natural to that species—Fact
3. Desiring to act is natural to *homo sapiens*—1, 2
4. People value what is natural to them—Assertion
5. What people value they wish to protect—Assertion
6. All people wish to protect their ability to act beyond all else—1, 3, 4, 5
7. The strongest interpersonal "oughts" are expressed via our highest value systems: religion, morality, and aesthetics—Assertion
8. All people must agree, upon pain of logical contradiction, that what is natural and desirable to them individually is natural and desirable to everyone collectively and individually—Assertion
9. Everyone must seek personal protection for her own ability to act via religion, morality, and/or aesthetics—6, 7
10. Everyone upon pain of logical contradiction must admit that all other humans will seek personal protection of their ability to act via religion, morality, and/or aesthetics—8, 9
11. All people must agree, upon pain of logical contradiction, that since the attribution of the Basic Goods of Agency are predicated generally, that it is inconsistent to assert idiosyncratic preferences—Fact
12. Goods that are claimed through generic predication apply equally to each agent and everyone has a stake in their protection—10, 11
13. Rights and duties are correlative—Assertion
14. Everyone has at least a moral right to the Basic Goods of Agency, and others in the society have a duty to provide those goods to all—12, 13

6. The entire listing is what Boylan calls the Table of Embeddedness (2004, ch. 3). It is as follows:

BASIC GOODS

Level One: *Most Deeply Embedded* (That which is absolutely necessary for Human Action)
Food, Clothing, Shelter, Protection from Unwarranted bodily harm
Level Two: *Deeply Embedded* (That which is necessary for effective basic action within any given society)

- Literacy in the language of the country
- Basic mathematical skills
- Other fundamental skills necessary to be an effective agent in that country, e.g., in the United States some computer literacy is necessary
- Some familiarity with the culture and history of the country in which one lives
- The assurance that those you interact with are not lying to promote their own interests
- The assurance that those you interact with will recognize your human dignity (as per above) and not exploit you as a means only

- Basic human rights such as those listed in the U.S. Bill of Rights and the United Nations Universal Declaration of Human Rights

SECONDARY GOODS

Life Enhancing: *Medium to High-Medium on Embeddedness*
- Basic Societal Respect
- Equal Opportunity to Compete for the Prudential Goods of Society
- Ability to pursue a life plan according to the Personal Worldview Imperative
- Ability to participate equally as an agent in the Shared Community Worldview Imperative

Useful: *Medium to Low-Medium Embeddedness*
- Ability to utilize one's real and portable property in the manner she chooses
- Ability to gain from and exploit the consequences of one's labor regardless of starting point
- Ability to pursue goods that are generally owned by most citizens, e.g., in the United States today a telephone, television, and automobile would fit into this class

Luxurious: *Low Embeddedness*
- Ability to pursue goods that are pleasant even though they are far removed from action and from the expectations of most citizens within a given country, e.g., in the United States today a European vacation would fit into this class
- Ability to exert one's will so that she might extract a disproportionate share of society's resources for her own use

WORKS CITED

Alker, H., Jr. 1965. *Mathematics and politics.* New York: Macmillan.

American Hospital Association. http://www.hospitalconnect.com (accessed December 19, 2005).

Andrulis, D. P., and L. M. Duchon. 2005. *Hospital care in the 100 largest cities and their suburbs 1996–2002.* Princeton, NJ: Robert Wood Johnson Foundation.

Barnato, A. E., A. M. Garber, C. R. Kagay, and M. C. McClellan. 1999. Trends in the use of intensive procedures at the end of life. In *Frontiers in health policy research*, vol. 2, ed. A. Garber. Cambridge, MA: MIT University Press.

Beauchamp, T. L., and J. F. Childress. 2001. *Principles of biomedical ethics*. 5th ed. New York: Oxford University Press.

Boylan, M. 2000. *Basic ethics.* Upper Saddle River, NJ: Prentice Hall.

———. 2004. *A just society.* Lanham, MD, and Oxford: Rowman & Littlefield.

Hester, D. M. 2001. Rethinking the residency matching process and questioning the value of competition in medicine. *Academic Medicine* 76 (4): 345–47.

———. 2003. What constitutes a "just" match?: A reply to Murphy. *Cambridge Quarterly of Healthcare Ethics* 12 (1): 78–82.

Hohfeld, W. 1919. *Fundamental legal conceptions.* New Haven, CT: Yale University Press.

King, M. L., Jr. 1963/1995. Letter from Birmingham Jail. In *Philosophy of Law*, 5th ed., ed. J. Feinberg. Belmont, CA: Wadsworth.

Lindquist, C. H. 1999. Health behind bars: Utilization and evaluation of medical care among jail inmates. *Journal of Community Health* 24 (2): 285–303.

Lubtiz, J. D., and G. F. Riley. 1993. Trends in Medicare payments in the last year of life. *New England Journal of Medicine* 328 (15): 1092–96.

Plato. 1903. *Republic* and *Gorgias*. Vols. 3 and 4 in *Platonis opera*, ed. J. Burnet. Oxford: Clarendon Press.

Provident Hospital of Cook County website: http://www.cookcountyresearch.net/prov.html (accessed December 19, 2005).

Scitovsky. 1984. The high cost of dying: What do the data show? *Milbank* 62 (4): 591–608.

———. 1994. The high cost of dying revisited. *Milbank* 72 (4): 561–91.

Stroger, J. H. 2005. *Presidential address to the board of commissioners of Cook County*, January 5.

Weisman, J. 2005. Justices to review DeLay-led districting. *Washington Post*, December 13.

13

Taking the Lead in Developing Institutional Policies

David T. Ozar

KEY POINTS

1. Differentiate three types of hospital ethics committee (HEC) policy advice.
2. Differentiate and respond to practical questions about three stances that an HEC might take regarding policy advice: Receptivity, Advocacy, and Mandate.
3. Evaluate an HEC's learning needs in order to provide policy advice.
4. Evaluate and respond to practical questions about an HEC's relation to an existing or proposed organizational ethics committee or compliance committee.

For most HECs, providing policy advice is understood to be part of the committee's mission along with clinical ethics case consulting and education. Such advice might relate to the clinical policies within the institution, but it is obvious that many of a healthcare institution's nonclinical policies have ethical import. Financial, employment, and many other business management policies, as well as policies regarding professional and educational matters, all have ethical issues embedded in them. So the possibility of an HEC making a contribution to the development of institutional policies, both clinical and nonclinical, deserves detailed consideration.

This chapter will identify three types of policy advice, namely clinical policy advice and two types of nonclinical policy advice. It will then consider three possible stances that an HEC might take toward advising: Receptivity, Advocacy, and Mandate. Each of these stances has educational implications for the HEC, and these implications will be discussed in the following sections. The final sections look at the relations of HECs to organizational ethics committees and compliance committees and propose some strategies that an HEC might pursue if its concern about policy matters suggests it should be involved in advocacy or should be seeking a mandate to provide policy advice. A brief bibliography of the literature on organizational ethics concludes the essay.

THREE TYPES OF POLICY ADVICE

While these divisions overlap, there are three types of policy advice in which an HEC might be involved: clinical policy advising, the application and interpretation of nonclinical policies, and creation of nonclinical policies.

The first kind of policy advice comes naturally to an HEC that is already engaged in clinical ethics consultation about cases, for it is not uncommon that a case in which the HEC has provided consultation assistance on clinical-ethical matters also raises a question about clinical policy either for the whole hospital or system, such as a DNR policy or a policy about the process for requesting organs for transplant, or for a particular clinical unit of the hospital, for example, a policy about the impact of a patient's DNR order on anesthesiologists during surgery or a policy on the purchase of ova by the fertility clinic.

When members of the HEC notice that a consultation raises a clinical policy question, then the HEC will need to decide whether it should wait either until some hospital or some system or relevant unit leader asks the HEC for assistance (which is the stance called "Receptivity" in the next section), or the HEC should be proactive in trying to get the policy question addressed ("Advocacy"). Of course, one could also imagine an institution where clinical policy matters, whether new policies or changes in previous ones, are required to be reviewed and evaluated for their ethical import by the HEC ("Mandate"). These three stances and HEC strategies in relation to them are addressed below.

Whatever the HEC's stance regarding clinical policy advising, it is important to distinguish the activity of drafting a policy's language and the thought process in which alternative candidates for a clinical policy on some matter are weighed and compared. When, for example, the hospital's clinical leadership or the leadership of a particular clinical unit asks the HEC for assistance in developing a policy, ordinarily they are also asking for assistance in wording it properly, and they may not differentiate between the two tasks in their request. Thus the development of proper wording is often the mechanism by which the HEC (or any other advisory body) offers its assistance in developing clinical policy. But this distinction can have practical importance if hospital or unit leadership comes to the HEC with a policy already determined, in need of drafting assistance only.

The characteristic that differentiates this first type of HEC policy advising from the two that follow is the specifically clinical nature of the policies advised on, namely, the applicability of clinical policies to treatment decisions; caregiver relations to patients, families, and each other; or other bedside, OR, ER, and similar decisions by caregivers. Note, however, that the most obvious marker of a clinical matter—the presence of just one patient receiving care—is absent here because what is being discussed is advice about policy, that is, it applies to a general class of patients or clinical situations. This is why the boundary between this type of policy advice and the two nonclinical types that follow is often blurry.

A second possible type of HEC involvement in institutional policy is HEC advice on the application and interpretation of a nonclinical institutional policy. Obviously, many institutional policy matters that are decided by nonclinical decision makers have significant impact on patients, caregivers, and others with whom the hospital or system deals and therefore raise important ethical questions. If the existence and the clinical ethics consulting role of the HEC are well publicized and are respected within the institution, nonclinical decision makers might decide to seek the committee's help on an ethically difficult matter. Suppose, for example, that the public relations office asks the HEC to evaluate the ethical implications of a particular print or media ad for the hospital or system, or the ethics of a proposed component of the institution's contract with its physicians' practice group is brought to the HEC for ethical evaluation by a negotiator for one side or the other.

Structurally, the way an HEC would provide assistance in such situations might well be identical to how the HEC structures its clinical ethics case consultations. But there are two important differences.

Obviously, first, the subject matter of these "consultations" is something nonclinical. Second, because administrative and managerial decisions in a formal organization like a hospital or health system typically have the weight of precedent for future issues of the same sort—no matter how particular and individualized the issue might be at the time—these decisions often impact future institutional decisions in a more significant way than the sorts of questions typically addressed in a clinical ethics case consultation.

In this second type of HEC involvement in policy advising, it is possible that the request for advice comes to the HEC by a nonclinical decision maker voluntarily seeking the HEC's advice, and the HEC has the option of responding or not, depending on its view of its own expertise in the matter. This is the stance called "Receptivity" in the next section. Or the HEC might contact a decision maker or nonclinical unit of the institution in order to offer its advice on how the policy should be interpreted or applied without having been asked ("Advocacy"). Or the institution could require that the HEC be consulted in interpreting and applying certain institutional policies ("Mandate").

In the third type of HEC involvement in policy, the HEC is directly involved in judging what nonclinical policies the institution should have in place in some matter, not just assisting nonclinical decision makers in interpreting and applying policies already created. Of course, the HEC's role would be to evaluate potential policies from an ethical point of view only, so an HEC would never be functioning alone in creating institutional policies.

Here again, the stance of the HEC may be that it will play such a role only when asked to by institutional policy makers (Receptivity). Or an HEC may determine that it should actively work for the creation of certain nonclinical institutional policies (Advocacy). It is possible that an institution would accord significant power to a HEC to advise on, craft, or even have veto power over proposed nonclinical policies from the perspective of the committee's ethics expertise. Some religiously affiliated hospitals and health systems, for example, accord significant responsibility of this sort to their "Mission-Ethics Committee," which may in some cases be the clinical HEC for the institution as well.

Some hospitals and systems have a committee that is distinct from the clinical HEC to provide ethics advice on nonclinical policy matters, and ideally on ethical questions in the conduct of the organization as a whole. It will therefore be important to discuss the rela-

tionships between an HEC and such "organizational ethics committees" and "compliance committees."

THREE STANCES: RECEPTIVITY, ADVOCACY, MANDATE

There are three stances that an HEC might adopt in regard to providing policy advice. All three are possible stances for an HEC providing clinical policy advice, and most HECs will have reflected on
them in connection to clinical policies. However, many HECs have
had little or no experience offering either type of nonclinical policy
advice. For these HECs, determining the best stance for the HEC to
take regarding nonclinical policy advice will be an important decision. Therefore, the remainder of this chapter will focus on providing advice on nonclinical policy, that is, the second and third types
of policy advice identified in the previous section.

First, an HEC may be Receptive, and only receptive, to its institution's policy makers seeking the HEC's assistance on a matter of nonclinical policy. Such an HEC responds with policy advice when asked
for it, but doesn't propose or advocate for new policies or for changes
in policy unless asked. (As indicated, one could imagine an HEC that
declined to offer ethics assistance on nonclinical matters even when
asked to do so. This fourth possible stance will not be discussed further here beyond saying that acting in this way once or twice would
almost certainly eliminate all future opportunity to become involved
in the institution's nonclinical policy making and might also have an
significant negative impact on its being involved in clinical policy advising.)

Secondly, an HEC's stance may be one of Advocacy, choosing to be
more proactive about raising nonclinical policy issues in general, or
in certain areas of special concern to the HEC. This stance admits of
many variations. For example, an HEC may advocate for a new or
changed nonclinical policy by proposing the idea to a relevant institutional leader or committee, but refrain from more active advocacy
once that has been done. Or an HEC may see itself as ethically required to advocate more actively, for example, by representing the
need for the policy or change to numerous institutional leaders or
committees or by repeated advocacy efforts about it. An HEC may
advocate only by direct personal contact, or it may produce reports
recommending new or changed policy in detailed terms, or it may

actually draft the policy it is advocating and offer the draft to those in relevant decision-making positions. An HEC might choose to engage in its advocacy through seeking the support of leaders or committees of the professional staff, or of particular senior administrators, or of other sources of influence within (or possibly even beyond) the institution, and so on.

Third, an HEC's stance in contributing to nonclinical institutional policy may be one of formal Mandate. In one form, a formal step of seeking the HEC's input on relevant ethical issues might be part of the formal process of policy creation at certain levels in the chain of command or for certain kinds of policies, or possibly across the board. On the other hand, the HEC might simply be the mandated "place to go" for ethics advice whenever an administrator or manager wanted it, but institutional decision makers might not be required to seek the committee's advice in any particular matter. In either case, as noted, since the HEC's stance in relation to nonclinical policy making is one of Mandate, with the implication that the committee's ability to decline to be of assistance, for lack of expertise or any other reason, would likely be limited.

EDUCATIONAL IMPLICATIONS

The Receptive stance will almost always mean that the HEC will have little impact on nonclinical institutional policy making. The work of administrators and managers is intense enough, and their habitual convictions that they are good people who are working in accord with the institution's mission and core values are ordinarily strong enough that few will consciously avert with any regularity to the need for additional ethics advice on a policy matter that is within their responsibility. Moreover, when they do see a need for ethics advice, they will typically ask assistance of another administrator or manager rather than someone outside the relevant leadership circle. One additional reason for this is that, if managers and administrators are even aware of the existence of the HEC and its ethics consulting role, they will typically see its function as narrowly clinical, rather than as including relevant ethical awareness of the challenges of good management and institutional policy.

Thus the only policy issues likely to be brought to an HEC that chooses the Receptive stance are clinical policy issues coming to the committee from clinical leaders within the institution. Educationally, this is good news. The HEC's clinical ethics background and its members' likely familiarity with how clinical policies are created within and impact the institution will almost always be sufficient for the HEC's needs in advising about clinical policy without a steep learning curve.

But it is worth pointing out that, if an HEC chooses to become an advocate for nonclinical policy matters, it cannot do so in good conscience without addressing the question of how it will obtain the relevant expertise. That is, the educational implications of an HEC moving beyond Receptivity are significant, and an HEC should not make this move without taking these implications seriously.

Regarding the second stance, Advocacy, an educational advantage is that the HEC can choose to exercise advocacy only in those nonclinical areas in which it either already has or can readily get the expertise it needs in order to advocate from an appropriate base of technical and institutional information. Obviously, any HEC that chooses to advocate for new or changed policies in a nonclinical area, but does so on the basis of poor information or a naive grasp of the issues involved, will quickly close the doors of the institution's decision makers to its assistance in nonclinical matters, and it might run the risk of jeopardizing its contribution to clinical matters as well.

If there is a Mandate that the HEC provide ethics assistance in the creation of nonclinical policy, then the HEC clearly has a serious responsibility to educate its members in relevant ways, seek assistance from experts outside the committee, and consider expanding its membership to include relevant expertise as well.

The HEC's education for such roles obviously needs to include the technical information needed to judge policy proposals in whatever particular area of policy is being considered and a detailed understanding of the institutional decision-making structures by which such policies are proposed, developed, and approved. In addition, and more subtly, the HEC also needs to educate itself in two foundational subject areas of this kind of ethics advising.

First, the committee needs to educate itself in the basic presuppositions of organizational ethics, that is, examination of ethical questions focused on the conduct of an organization as a whole. There is a strong tendency in American culture to view corporations and other larger organizations very impersonally, as if they were complex machines, and as if the only values and goals and therefore the only standards of conduct involved in them were the values and goals and standards of the individual persons who run them and work in them. But the perspective needed here views organizations as having values and goals, as capable of conduct that is appropriate or inappropriate, ethical or unethical.

Therefore, the HEC needs to educate itself about what is presupposed when one views an organization as a unitary actor capable of acting ethically or unethically, and to understand what can and cannot be reasonably said of an institutional actor of this sort. The HEC needs to examine the role of mission and core institutional values in the activity of any organization, and also the standing of such organizational values within the broader realm of ethical reflection and judgment. It also needs to consider the relation of these institutional standards of an organization's conduct to the judgments and actions of the individuals playing specific roles, especially senior decision-making roles, within the organization.

Second, the HEC needs to ask the same questions with regard to the HEC's own institution. The committee needs to have a detailed knowledge of the organization's actual mission and core values—and of the connection between these, whether closer or more remote, and what the institution tells the public about itself in its formal self-descriptions and its public relations documents. It must learn about how this mission and these core values are, or are not, lived out in the work and practice of the various departments and units of the organization, and especially how they impact the decisions of managers and administrators in various areas of institutional decision making. All ethical reflection at the organizational level must take account of the mission and core values as ordinarily the principal determinants of right conduct for the organization, even though these standards themselves need to be regularly examined from a broader ethical point of view.

LEARNING ORGANIZATIONAL ETHICS

The field of organizational ethics, as a subfield within healthcare ethics, has grown significantly in the last decade, and there are a number of books, journal articles, and other resources to assist the HEC in this process. A survey of these resources will be offered in the final section of this essay. There are also a number of scholars in the healthcare ethics community whom an interested HEC could call on to provide educational programs or guidance as the committee prepared itself for this role and, in special circumstances, as it wrestled with a particular issue or policy. In addition, there is much in the literature of the business ethics community that will be helpful to those interested in self-education in this area, especially the literature of what is called "Stakeholder Theory," that will be very helpful in articulating the relation of organizational mission and core values to the organization's impact on the wide array of persons whom it affects.

There is also a sizable body of literature by scholars in organization theory, both in general and in the specialty area of organization theory that focuses on healthcare organizations, that addresses the role and impact of institutional mission and core values in such organizations. Finally, there is a sizable literature in systems theory that is relevant to understanding how organizations work and the role of the values and commitments of component parts of institutions in relation to its judgments and conduct as a whole.

While it may be thoroughly obvious, it seems worth mentioning that an HEC's self-education in organizational ethics and relevant technical and institutional matters will almost certainly not happen if the group does not agree to formal educational activities. These can be study groups about relevant literature or workshops or retreats. They can be led by members of the committee who already have some expertise or who educate themselves to do so, or the committee can engage outside experts to assist. It is possible that these educational activities might be squeezed into the committee's regular meetings, but if the committee is already active in its clinical work of consultation and education, then almost certainly the committee will not educate itself adequately for nonclinical policy advising unless it makes additional time outside of its regular meetings.

RELATING TO ORGANIZATIONAL ETHICS COMMITTEES

As the importance of examining institutional policies from the point of view of the mission and core values of the whole organization has been increasingly recognized within healthcare institutions, a few have established ethics committees with this as their specific perspective, distinct from the committee that does clinical ethics consultations and other clinical ethics work in the organization. Such a

committee may have any number of formal names and locations in
the chain of command, especially because the term "ethics" has a
way of putting some people off. There is also a fear on the part of
some senior administrators that such a committee may be used inappropriately by others if not carefully limited in its mandate and
even more importantly in how it is viewed in the organization. The
Joint Commission on the Accreditation of Healthcare Organizations
has begun to look for evidence of an organization's awareness of organizational ethics issues during its surveys in recent years. Therefore, as organizations seek to make such evidence clear and concrete,
the interest in having a distinct organizational ethics committee may
grow stronger.

As mentioned, if no such committee exists, but a need is seen for
ethics advising on nonclinical policy matters, this task may well fall
to the HEC if its clinical work is respected within the institution. But
the question to address here is how an HEC should relate to such a
separate organizational ethics committee where one exists.

The short answer, obviously, is collegially. Where organizational
committees as distinct entities have been created, their members are
usually representatives of the senior administrative offices of the institution, for example, finance, legal, public relations, human relations, and patient care management. It is important that the HEC
and the organizational ethics committee work well together, especially because there is no clear line dividing clinical policy and nonclinical policy in a healthcare institution. Therefore, it is important
that there be persons who are members of both committees to assure
clarity of communication between them and a continuing collegial
distribution of tasks between them, as well as mutual consultation
on issues that concern them both. Each ought to feel comfortable referring issues to the other when they are also in its purview and in
advising the other and seeking the other's advice.

But it is also important that each one have a clear range of responsibility that is distinct from the other, even though many issues may
overlap. This is something that should be formally articulated, to the
extent possible, because it cannot be fully resolved simply by the two
parties' commitment to collegiality. It is, in other words, a substantive
matter, not merely a procedural one, and it is best negotiated in advance to begin with, and then by appropriate adjustment as ambigu-
ities arise. For the same reason, it will be best if neither of these committees reports to the other in the chain of command, but rather if

both report directly or indirectly to the same senior officer or committee. That is, neither should be subordinate to the other because the real difference in their roles is a difference in substantive subject matter, and their institutional relationship should be designed to preserve this as what differentiates them. Currently, in a number of institutions, the HEC reports to the compliance committee (ideally with some measure of shared membership). If there was also a distinct organizational ethics committee in such an institution, having it also report to the compliance committee would seem best.

Where an organizational ethics committee exists or is created, in other words, the HEC should work hard to clarify and differentiate the roles of the two entities. In such a situation, almost certainly, the HEC should not engage in any ethics-policy advising about nonclinical matters that happen to be brought to it, but should refer them to the organizational ethics committee. This is the only situation in which the stance of referring all nonclinical matters elsewhere would seem appropriate; the HEC should be involved in nonclinical policy advising in this situation only at the request of the other committee.

COMPLIANCE COMMITTEES

Although other names are to be found, most health systems and independent hospitals now have a committee called the compliance committee (since the motivation for institutions to create such a committee derives from the law, most organizations simply use this title, with its legal connotations). Some institutions that have a compliance committee have created it without involving the institution's HEC in the process in any way—much less seeking its advice about the matter—because the functions of the compliance committee and the functions of an HEC may be thought to be clearly distinct from one another.

The work of a compliance committee typically includes preparation and dissemination the organization's code of conduct for employees. But its chief responsibility is to make sure at a very high level of decision making within the organization that everything it does is in conformity with the myriad legal regulations affecting healthcare institutions, especially billing, coding, and related fiscal matters. Therefore an entity focused on ethics in the clinical setting, especially in regard to treatment decisions and relations between caregivers and patients, families, and one another, namely the HEC as it is usually understood, seems to be concerned with a different area of the institution's life altogether.

To understand this view of the distance between the two committees' tasks, it will be helpful to review a little history related to compliance committees, specifically the revision of the Federal Sentencing Guidelines for Organizations that became effective in November 1991.

In contrast to the previous document used by federal judges in sentencing an organization found guilty of violating federal laws and regulations, the revised guidelines provide that the basic sentence of a convicted organization is to be either multiplied (as much as fourfold) or mitigated (by as much as 95 percent), according to the organization's demonstrated record of working to monitor and minimize wrongdoing by its employees and of accepting responsibility, cooperating with law enforcement officials, and self-reporting of an offense. According to the *Federal Ethics Report* (Nov. 1995, 5), of the 208 organizations found guilty and sentenced under the guidelines from November 1991 to June 1995, only one company's record was sufficiently strong to have its sentence mitigated by reason of an effective program of compliance with the guidelines. But 87 percent of them did receive some credit, especially for accepting responsibility, cooperation, or self-reporting.

Due diligence under the guidelines has been summarized under these seven headings:

1. Establish compliance standards that address potential criminal conduct specifically relevant to the organization's business operations;
2. Establish a formal structure for the compliance program that includes a high-level officer assigned responsibility for the program;
3. Build a system to avoid delegation of substantial discretionary authority to known wrongdoers;
4. Communicate the compliance standards effectively to all employees;
5. Develop effective measures of compliance and of the communication of standards to the organization through monitoring, effective audits, and confidential internal reporting mechanisms (for example, a hotline);

6. Develop a fair and effective enforcement mechanism to ensure discipline;
7. Respond appropriately to detected offenses and investigations thereof.

For a number of organizations, consent decrees and plea agreements have imposed comprehensive compliance programs that have added specific court-mandated policies, procedures, and systems to the guidelines' basic due diligence criteria. So obviously, there is a lot at stake here for any organization dealing with the federal government, and that includes any organization that accepts Medicare payments.

This is why most healthcare institutions have appointed a "chief compliance officer" and established a compliance committee to assist that person in his or her job. This is why the central focus of this officer and this committee is on making sure the organization is in conformity with relevant laws and regulations and why so many institutions see their compliance committees as performing a very different function from an HEC.

While most healthcare organizations have formed compliance committees, there are two additional facts about the Federal Sentencing Guidelines that HEC members should be aware of. The first is that nonprofit organizations are not presently liable to the application of the guidelines as for-profit entities are. The second is a Supreme Court ruling in January 2005, *Booker v. US*, that the guidelines as previously interpreted were unconstitutional because, when applying them to organizations, judges used them to enhance defendant organizations' sentences on the basis of information that had not been presented to a jury. As a result, the Federal Sentencing Guidelines have now become just that, "guidelines" for judges rather than mandatory sentencing ranges. But neither of these facts has lessened the importance of having an effective compliance committee in the life of most healthcare institutions.

Many organizations that have a compliance committee believe that they therefore already have in place a committee with the task of looking at how well it carries out its mission and core values. That is, in many organizations, the compliance committee is thought to be an organizational ethics committee, even though providing advice about organizational ethics (in any of the three stances) is not typically part of the work of such a compliance committee.

So even with a well-designed and efficient compliance committee in place, an HEC may conclude that the ethical aspects of important nonclinical policies are not being carefully examined anywhere within the institution. The question faced by an HEC under such circumstances is much more complex than it would be if there were no compliance committee, because senior administration may well believe a great deal of resources have already been spent to establish a formal entity to address ethical issues at the organizational level. Like many other questions faced by an HEC concerned about the ethics of its institution's nonclinical policies, this is a question requiring careful strategic thinking.

STRATEGIES

There are no algorithms for strategy. The various paths mentioned above by which an HEC interested in Advocacy might proceed can serve only as examples of what might be the best way to proceed in practice to enhance an HEC's role in nonclinical policy formation.

Two points are most important in this: first, in working for institutional change, there are no substitutes for careful strategic thinking in advance of action, for solid facts and careful realism about likely outcomes, and for the patience that these all require. Simply being certain that a certain change in policy will make life better for many people and that the proposed policy is far superior to any available alternative does not mean that those with decision-making power will be similarly impressed. Institutions, by their very nature, create parameters within which senior (and all other) decision makers operate, and careful strategic thinking is necessary (even as it is, under the name of "tact," in person-to-person relations) to get anything worthwhile done. Second, an HEC's strategies must themselves be carefully examined from a broad ethical point of view. In particular, the effect of an HEC initiative must be weighed carefully from every angle. Sometimes what would most efficiently move an HEC's institutional initiative forward will so compromise the institution's perception of the HEC as a source of balanced ethical wisdom, or will so weaken the HEC's ability to seek support in other matters from a particular administrator or committee, or in some other way damage the HEC's ability to do its work in the future, that other means may need to be identified to achieve the goal at hand, even if they are less efficient or less likely of success in the short run.

While admitting that there are no algorithms for strategy, the single most important strategy for an HEC that hopes to contribute an ethics perspective to the development of nonclinical institutional policy has already been described. It is self-education by the HEC—both the general education in organizational ethics that will enable the committee to have a coherent framework and set of concepts and relevant ethics vocabulary to use in making its case, and the particular education it needs about its own institution's mission, core values, and decision-making structures so that its case is matched to what the institution and its senior decision makers can hear. Third, the HEC needs education, whether acquired directly by the members of the committee themselves or with the help of other experts, so that the committee's ethical judgments about policies are based on good information or a sophisticated understanding of what is at stake. If an HEC's judgments and proposals do not have this level of expertise as their foundation, all of the skillful strategy in the world is unlikely to save them.

An HEC that is active and has become skilled in providing ethics advice on clinical matters through clinical ethics case consultations, advice on clinical policy, and clinical ethics education should probably consider whether there is a need for it to become more active in contributing an ethics perspective to the development of nonclinical policy in its institution. Answering this question will require careful reflection on what other committees and structures are in place in the institution, especially if there is a compliance committee or an organizational ethics committee. The HEC will need to determine if it has the time and is willing to commit the effort to undertake such a task with care, and especially if it is willing to educate itself as much as will be necessary in order to do the job properly and have realistic hope of being effective.

As mentioned at the outset, most HECs affirm that providing policy advice is part of the committee's mission along with clinical ethics case consulting and education. But in practice, this function seems to be carried out by most HECs only in relation to clinical policy, a task for which most mature HECs are well prepared. The harder question and the greater challenge is whether, when, and how an HEC should offer ethics advice to enhance the institution's nonclinical policy making. This chapter has aimed to provide HECs with a summary of the questions they ought be asking themselves as they consider this possibility.

FOR FURTHER REFLECTION

1. Which types of policy advice, if any, does your HEC provide within your institution and to whom?
2. What is your HEC's stance in providing these types of policy advice?
3. Do you believe your HEC's stance is the best stance for it to take at this point in its life in the institution? Why or why not? If not, what stance would be better and why? If some stance would be better, is there a practical way for the HEC to begin to move in that direction?
4. What are your HEC's most important learning needs if it is to undertake more policy advice work in the institution?
5. What is your HEC's relation to the organizational ethics committee, if any, or the compliance committee in your institution? Is this the best relation for your HEC to have at this time in its life in the institution? Why or why not? If not, what relation would be better and why? If some relation would be better, is there a practical way for the HEC to begin to move in that direction?

ADDITIONAL RESOURCES

American College of Healthcare Executives. *Code of ethics*. Available at http://www.ache.org.

American Society for Bioethics and Humanities. *Annual meetings of the ASBH organizational ethics affinity group*. See Affinity Group website at: www.asbh.org.

Boyle, P. J., E. R. DuBose, S. J. Ellingson, D. E. Guinn, and D. B. McCurdy. 2001. *Organizational ethics in health care: Principles, cases, and practical solutions*. San Francisco: Jossey-Bass.

Collins, J., and J. Porras. 1994/1997. *Built to last: Successful habits of visionary companies*. New York: Harper-Collins.

Darr, K. 1997. *Ethics in health services management*. 3rd ed. Baltimore: Health Professions Press.

Fiorelli, P., and C. Rooney. *Federal sentencing guidelines: A guide for internal auditors*. Altamonte Springs, FL: The Institute of Internal Auditors.

Freeman, R. E. 1999. Stakeholder theory and the modern corporation. Reprinted in *Ethical issues in business*, 6th ed., ed. T. Donaldson and P. H. Werhane, 247–57. Upper Saddle River, NJ: Prentice-Hall.

Hall, R. T. 2000. *An introduction to healthcare organizational ethics.* New York: Oxford University Press.

Hosmer, L. 1996. *The ethics of management.* 3rd ed. Boston: Irwin/McGraw-Hill.

Kaptein, M. 1998. *Ethics management: Auditing and developing the ethical content of organizations.* Dordrecht/Boston: Kluwer Academic Publishers.

Khushf, G. 1997. Administrative and organizational ethics. *HEC Forum* 9:299–309.

McDaniel, C. 2004. *Organizational ethics: Research and ethical environments.* Burlington, VT: Ashgate.

Metzger, M., D. R. Dalton, and J. W. Hill. 1993. The organization of ethics and the ethics of organizations: The case for expanded organizational ethics audits. *Business Ethics Quarterly* 3 (1): 27–43.

Mills, A. E., E. M. Spencer, and P. H. Werhane. 2001. *Developing organization ethics in healthcare: A case-based approach to policy, practice, and compliance.* Hagerstown, MD: University Publishing Group.

Organizational Ethics: Healthcare, Business, and Policy. Hagerstown, MD: University Publishing Group. An interdisciplinary journal on healthcare organizations and their ethics.

O'Toole, B. 1994. *A social contract foundation for the professional ethics of health care administrators.* PhD dissertation, Loyola University, Chicago.

Ozar, D. T. 2004. The gold standard for ethics education and effective decision-making in health care organizations. *Organizational Ethics: Healthcare, Business, and Policy* 1 (1): 32–42.

Ozar, D. T., et al. 2000. *Organizational ethics in health care: A framework for ethical decision-making by provider organizations.* Chicago: American Medical Association Institute of Ethics. Available at http://www.ama-assn.org/ama/upload/mm/369/organizationalethics.pdf.

Payne, L. S. 1994. Managing for organizational integrity. *Harvard Business Review* 72 (2): 106–17.

———. 1997. *Leadership, ethics, and organizational integrity.* Chicago: Irwin.

———. 2003. *Value shift: Why companies must merge social and financial imperatives to achieve superior performance.* New York: McGraw-Hill.

Pearson, S., J. Sabin, and E. Emanuel. 2003. *No margin, no mission.* New York: Oxford University Press.

Potter, R. L., ed. 1999. Special issue on organizational ethics. *Journal of Clinical Ethics* 10 (3): 171–246.

Reiser, S. J. 1994. The ethical life of health care organizations. *Hastings Center Report* 24 (6): 28–35.

Scott, W. R. 1998. *Organizations: Rational, natural, and open systems.* Upper Saddle River, NJ: Prentice-Hall.

Spencer, E., A. Mills, M. Rorty, and P. H. Werhane. 2000. *The ethics of healthcare organizations.* New York: Oxford University Press.

U.S. Department of Justice, *Sentencing organizations, federal sentencing guidelines.* Available at http://www.ussc.gov/guide/ch8web.htm.

U.S. Sentencing Commission. 1991. Sentencing guidelines for organizational defendants. *Federal Register* 56:22786–22797.

Weber, L. J. 2001. *Business ethics in healthcare: Beyond compliance*. Bloomington: Indiana University Press.

Werhane, P. H. 1991. The ethics of healthcare as a business. *Business and Professional Ethics Journal* 9 (3–4): 7–20.

Werhane, P. H., and M. V. Rorty. 2000. Special section on organizational ethics. *Cambridge Quarterly of Healthcare Ethics* 9 (2): 145–241.

Wicks, A., ed. 2002. Special issue on health care and business ethics. *Business Ethics Quarterly* 12 (4): 409–526.

Worthley, J. A. 1999. *Organizational ethics in the compliance context*. Chicago: Health Administration Press.

14

Handling the Law in HEC Deliberations

Kenneth A. De Ville and Gregory L. Hassler

KEY POINTS

1. Historical evolution of hospital ethics committees (HECs)
2. Necessary synergy between the law and bioethics in HEC activities
3. Benefits and limitations of lawyers and legal perspectives on HECs

For three decades, HECs, clinicians, administrators, ethicists, and scholars have struggled with the relationship between bioethics and law and lamented what they view as the distracting and deleterious effect of law on HEC discussions, deliberations, and recommendations. On some HECs, "talk of law as well as lawyers may be banned from the ethical discussions" (Scott 2000). These concerns are frequently based on experience, reasonable fears, and the accurate observation that law and ethics are not always compatible. But despite these concerns, legal considerations are frequently difficult or impossible to ignore. While all bioethical questions do not inevitably express themselves as well as legal questions, the common subject matter of the two endeavors and the parallels between ethical and legal reasoning suggest that HECs will never completely escape the influence and consideration of the law. Nor should they try. Law played a key role in the birth and the proliferation of HECs. Law and

legal thinking have contributed as well to the intellectual content
and the procedural shape of bioethics discourse both within HECs
and without. Finally, accurate and thoughtful legal knowledge and
judgments are irreplaceable parts of HECs' practical work within the
institution. These observations support neither the substitution of legal analysis for moral reasoning nor lawyers for ethicists. Instead, as
HECs become increasingly institutionalized and mature, they should
strive for a clear, sophisticated and integrated view of the relationship between law and their work.

PRESENT AT THE CREATION

Given the role that law, legal considerations, and legal and quasi-
legal institutions have played in the establishment and proliferation
of HECs, it is not surprising that law continues to play a central role
as well in the work and deliberations of HECs (Scott 2000; Wolf
1991; Annas 1991; Cranford and Doudera 1984; Hoffman 1991; Povar 1991; Wilson 1998). Many of the earliest and most important influences on HECs were legal or regulatory in nature. The Quinlan
case (1976), of course, cited a then-obscure law review article that
suggested that HECs could help oversee family and clinician requests
to discontinue life-sustaining treatment (Quinlan 1976). It soon became clear that courts would at least consider recommendations and
conclusions of HECs in their adjudication of problematic cases.
Saikewicz (1977), Spring (1980), and Torres (1984) implicitly or explicitly acknowledged the potential legal relevance of HEC deliberations and conclusions. Advocates of the HEC model have cited the
HEC's potential guidance to courts as a benefit of the institution and
as a spur to its growth (Wolf 1991). Moreover, the perhaps unfortunate hope that HECs would provide legal "cover" for individuals and
institutions making difficult decisions may have accelerated the mul-
tiplication of HECs (Annas 1991).

The 1983 President's Commission for the Study of Ethical Problems in Medicine represented an important "nonlegal" spur to the
growth of HECs (President's Commission 1983), however, legal influences and concerns continued to be important. The so-called
"Baby Doe Rules" (1984) ratified the use of "infant care review committees," introduced the HEC format into the healthcare institution
mainstream, and according to some observers, "may have the most

significant effect on the movement toward establishing ethics committees for all patients" (Cranford and Doudera 1984). Legally mandated institutional review boards have also influenced the introduction of the HEC format to healthcare institutions and helped pioneer the notion of HEC review of decisions and activities that were once left in the hands of physicians, researchers, patients, and subjects (Scott 2000). According to one report, the number of hospitals with HECs doubled from 1983 to 1985 (Povar 1991).

Several state legislatures promoted the use of HEC review in problematic cases. Maryland, in 1987, for instance, required the establishment of an "advisory committee" in each healthcare institution. (Hoffman 1991). Texas's 1999 medical futility and end-of-life decision-making legislation goes further and mandates HEC review under certain circumstances (Flamm 2000). New Jersey's administrative code requires hospitals to have either an HEC or a prognosis committee. Some states, such as Arizona, Hawaii, and Montana, do not require HECs, but legally support their activities by granting members qualified immunity from liability (Wilson 1998). In 1992, the Joint Commission on the Accreditation of Healthcare Organizations (JCAHO) required as part of the accreditation process that institutions provide mechanisms for dealing with the ethical issues that arise in health care (Powell 1998; Scott 2000). Many institutions attempted to meet this requirement by establishing or relying on HECs. JCAHO does not constitute a legal entity, but legal deference to JCAHO directives in a number of areas imbue JCAHO with a quasi-legal stature that makes it hard to ignore. Given that law is so intricately woven into the advent and growth of the HEC, it seems unrealistic to believe that it can be excluded from ethical deliberations. Law may also play at least an ancillary role when HECs serve as de facto facilitators or mediators in helping participants to sort through ethical conflicts and options for action.

LAW'S INFLUENCE ON BIOETHICS AND HEC DELIBERATIONS

Roger Dworkin has suggested that HECs' practical need for timely guidance has led some participants to rely on law instead of ethics, moral reasoning being viewed by some as a slow, cumbersome, and complicated way to reach answers already answered by the law

(Dworkin 1996). While Dworkin (1996) warns against an "unthinking" application of law to questions that cry out for the more nuanced analysis, he stresses that it would be "both stupid and unrealistic" to suggest that the law has no role to play in resolving the issues or in helping others resolve them through facilitation or mediation. The most appropriate posture is to recognize the place of the law, while realizing that its ability to answer bioethics questions will always be "severely limited" (Dworkin 1996).

But there are also a number of commentators who believe that law has shaped not only the developing of HECs, but of bioethics thought as well. George Annas, for example, boldly declares that "American law, not philosophy or medicine, is primarily responsible for the agenda, development and current state of American bioethics" (Annas 1993). He traces bioethics's predominantly rights-based approach and its propensity to decide cases by applying principles to facts in a systematic way to the pervasive influence of law in U.S. society. Similarly, according to Alexander Capron, law's influence on bioethics helps explain why the field tends to focus on "abstract principles" rather than "empirical findings," and on "proceduralism" rather than on "specific normative conclusions" (Capron 1999).

Moreover from *Baby Doe* to *Quinlan* to *Baby K*, the bioethics agenda and the HEC movement itself have been driven by high-profile legal cases (Capron 1999). According to Connie Zuckerman, "the law has been an active participant in these efforts to redefine our medical, moral and social commitments to dying patients and their families" (Zuckerman 1999). Similarly, the legal doctrine of informed consent, for example, has had, perhaps unfortunately, far more impact on the physician-patient relationship than the myriad of learned and insightful literature on the same topic (Brody 1989). As a result, a variety of bioethics debates take place in the pervasive "shadow" of the law either in their attempts to influence legal proceedings or to articulate legal principles or policy, whether it be in the form of legislation or institutional mandates (Capron 1999). For example, before healthcare institutions seek legal authorization to withdraw care in controversial scenarios, they frequently first choose to secure HEC ratification for their proposed actions. In the high-profile *Gilgunn, Wanglie*, and *Baby K* cases, the respective institutions first secured the counsel and approval of their HECs before attempting to remove life-sustaining treatment against the wishes of the patients' surrogate decision makers.

The intellectual pedigree of bioethics is not the topic of this chapter. The development of intellectual and social movements as complex as bioethics are far too seamless and holistic to winnow out the precise contributions of the various disciplines—especially two as closely allied as moral and legal reasoning. One might explain how any one of a dozen disciplines has made significant contributions to the bioethics endeavor. What remains important is that law has left and continues to leave an indelible mark on the practice of bioethics, and, consequently, on the conduct and deliberations of HECs. As importantly, the vast majority of HEC members have been steeped in a U.S. culture imbued with a constitutionally and legally based view of justice. These habits of mind are almost necessarily, albeit implicitly, carried into and made part of HEC discussions even if attempts are made scrupulously to avoid discussions of substantive law. Instead of attempting the impossible task of banishing all things law from bioethical discourse, HECs should recognize that their identities were formed and continue to be influenced by a multiplicity of factors. Maturity of individual HECs, as well as of the institution as a whole, will allow them to accept these various formative influences in such a way as to mitigate the negative and cultivate the positive.

HECS AND THE INESCAPABLE RELEVANCE OF LAW

But history and pedigree are not the only reasons that law does and should play a role in HEC deliberations. Given the inherently practical nature of the work of HECs, it would be irresponsible to completely banish law from ethics discussions. Bioethics as practiced in HECs is, first and foremost, an attempt to unravel the morally right choices in the context of specific clinical issues and the development of specific institutional practices and policies. The goal of such discussions is to provide guidance for clinical and institutional actions that will ultimately affect real, flesh and blood patients. The options explored in facilitation and mediation discussions must also meet the scrutiny of law. The pervasive nature of law in society and medicine means that the implementation of any decision or policy will also involve implicit and explicit legal considerations. There may, of course, be severe to modest legal penalties for individuals and institutions failing to follow relevant medical and legal guidance on a topic. But in addition, most individuals feel some sense of moral duty to obey the law and believe that it carries at least some moral weight in and of itself and beyond the potential negative consequences of abrogating it (Murphy and Coleman 1990). As a result, bioethical questions, at a practical level, almost inescapably involve questions of ethics *and* questions of law, which the HECs must confront, reconcile, or at least acknowledge. While it is true that what is ethical may differ from what is legal (or from the option that poses the fewest legal risks), this is not always the case. Indeed, in most cases, a clear and reasonable knowledge of the law will enable HECs, clinicians, and institutions to pursue the path they deem most ethical and clinically efficacious, while at the same time posing less risk. Accurate knowledge of the law can free clinical actors instead of tying their hands.

Thus, legal awareness can and in most cases *should* play a critical role in the deliberations and other activities of HECs. And, as a result, responsible HECs must have knowledge, or access to knowledge, regarding not only the relevant medical law, but how that law is likely to play out in a real-life scenario similar to that under consideration. Just as it is ethically imperative that HEC deliberations be conducted on the basis of accurate clinical information and scientific judgment, it is equally essential that HECs possess accurate information to help them assess legal issues in clinical situations and to take the most appropriate measures, and to aid the stakeholders in facilitating appropriate options.

HECs should have, through a committee member or resource, a detailed and nuanced understanding of the statutory and case law in the relevant jurisdiction applicable to the case or issue under consideration. While an exhaustive list of legal topics would be impossible to create, HECs deal with a set of fairly predictable range of issues on a regular basis. They might include the law related to:

advance directives
living wills
durable power(s) of attorney
surrogate decision makers
definition of death
"futility"/inappropriate care
organ donation
nutrition and hydration
DNRs

EMTALA
informed consent
confidentiality and privacy
reporting laws
professional liability
general liability (for example, personal injury, defamation, false
    imprisonment, etc.)
agency and vicarious liability
elder abuse
reproductive issues
competence and decision-making capacity
involuntary commitment/dangerousness
guardianship
Baby Doe regulations
age of majority/emancipated minors
minor consent to medical procedures
child abuse and neglect
parental rights
licensure and scope of practice
restraints
billing for medical care
abandonment and American Medical Association discharges
criminal law (for example, battery, homicide, etc.)
clinical trials research
local court structure

These reflect the range of legal issues that might surface in relatively routine HEC deliberations and other activities and might affect the analysis of the case, the available options considered by the committee, and the decisions or recommendations ultimately made by the group. HECs should have a member who can provide guidance on these issues or have access to consultative resources in a timely way.

But knowing the applicable so-called Black Letter law is not sufficient. HECs should understand as well the law in action, as it is practiced. The "law in action" includes an informed insight of how the relevant panoply of legal actors (judges, district attorneys, plaintiffs' attorneys, and so forth) typically or are likely to interpret and apply the legal provisions in question. While the content of the statutory law provides key insight into a legal requirement, the way that statute is interpreted and applied by judges is nearly as crucial. Such insight is especially important in scenarios in which legal risk, either civil or criminal, plays a role. In these situations, it is important as well to have a sense of what kind of factual scenario is likely to generate attention from a plaintiff's attorney or attorney general. While many legal actions are *theoretically* possible, the decision to sue an institution or individual civilly or to charge a physician criminally involves complicated judgment decisions based on a range of considerations. Finally, HEC discussions and activities must also be informed by some knowledge of the procedural realities of the legal world. Procedural realities frequently dictate whether a particular case will proceed. If a procedural barrier is likely to block an otherwise viable legal action, then the HECs' hopes or fears based only on consideration of the substantive law will not materialize. Knowledge of how the legal system or service operates in practice also aids in the fashioning of appropriate options. For example, an HEC member might in good faith assume that reporting an issue of child abuse or neglect to a department of social services will resolve the issue under discussion. However, familiarity with the actual operation of child protective services, as well as the written law regarding abuse and neglect, might refute that assumption and highlight the need to explore other solutions. In sum, the HEC should have access to a competent legal resource that will allow them to understand the law both in print and in context.

IN PRAISE OF LAW?

There are many ways in which legal perspectives can enrich and aid bioethical discussions. Law as a discipline and a body of knowledge is far from useless in the weighing of ethical options in medicine. Law has proved an effective discipline in the formal, institutionalized resolution of conflicts. It places a high premium on objectivity, impartiality, and consistency. Legal reasoning and argumentation are based on a vigorous and open debate of the alternatives of a position. It is a useful means, in some cases, of identifying weaknesses in opposing positions.

Law, moreover, is not devoid of moral content and may be relevant at least as a guide or articulation of the minimally accepted bounds of behavior. As Oliver Wendell Holmes noted, "The law is the witness and external deposit of our moral life. Its history is the history of the moral development of the race" (Holmes 1897). Despite Holmes's exaggerated contention, there are many ways in which he is correct. The President's Commission for the Study of Ethical Problems in Medicine recognized that "law is one of the basic means through which a society translates its values into policies and applies them to human conduct" (President's Commission 1983). Law *is*, in some ways, an illustrative collection of society's moral beliefs and attitudes, and for that reason, legal conclusions on biomedical issues are sometimes approximate reflections of ordinary moral reasoning.

In short, the relationship between law and bioethics is far more complicated than one discipline influencing another. It is one of mutuality; law informs bioethics, and bioethics informs the law. But more important, these and other disciplines likely share so many themes and traditions because they are all heirs to a common cultural, political, and intellectual heritage. These intellectual endeavors are interwoven in such a way as to make their disentanglement practically impossible. Law will continue to play a role in the moral deliberations of HECs because conceptually it is still difficult to separate the two in the American mind.

THE PERILS AND LIMITS OF LAW

Despite parallels between legal reasoning and moral problem solving, there are clear dis-analogies that highlight the limitations of a legal approach to ethical deliberations. In terms of substantive positions, law has been used to support slavery, involuntary sterilization, and discriminatory practices, as well as to delay ethical, socially beneficial, and just civil rights and social welfare programs. Sometimes legal reasoning is nothing more than the playing out of a relatively mechanical recurring set of arguments and counterarguments (Balkin 1986). To further its vaunted objectivity and consistency, legal process, training, and tradition have tended to downplay humanity and individuality in favor of the principles or doctrines involved. While this model is successful at achieving some limited goals, it may not be the appropriate model for resolving bioethical dilemmas. Finally, legal-style reasoning tends to focus ethical discussion on principles and on the relative rights of patient, physician, society, and institution. While these considerations are important, they may sometimes dilute equally or more important sources of ethical guidance.

Clearly, neither courtroom nor appellate law decisions guarantee a morally correct result. As the nineteenth-century legal adage recognizes, "Hard cases make bad law." Virtually all bioethics cases, at least those of the sort faced by HECs, represent hard cases, and it is arguable that there are numerous instances of "bad law" in biomedical jurisprudence. Legal decisions are subject to interest-group politics, the personal philosophy of judges and legislators, bad research, and sometimes poor lawyering. In addition, much law is the result of a particular case or situation presented for adjudication or remedy. A court's ruling on that case sometimes generates doctrine that is later applied to analogous situations. Therefore, the character of the cases originally presented to judges for adjudication may sometimes undermine the universality and utility of the resulting doctrine. Some scholars argue that while law is related to morality, it typically lags behind it (Hart 1961). As a result, sometimes law will not even serve as an accurate reflection of collected social wisdom, let alone as an objective, well-reasoned, reliable ethical guide for individual cases faced by an ethics committee (De Ville 1994). Ultimately, the interplay between law and ethics in bioethical deliberation, however, springs from the still-unsettled relationship between law and ethics in general. The fact that the nature of that interaction remains in dispute contributes to the continued uncertainty regarding the law's proper domain (Murphy and Coleman 1990).

The fear of liability has reached epidemic proportions not only among physicians but also across the entire gamut of healthcare professionals, including many members and potential members of the HEC. While concerns regarding liability are legitimate, a number of studies have found that many in the healthcare field significantly exaggerate the dangers of liability (De Ville 1998). These inflated fears can affect both clinical care and ethical discussions. Risk management concerns can preempt or distort ethical discussions and result in defensive postures or measures that threaten some risk of unnecessary harm, risk, discomfort, anxiety, inconvenience, or cost for the patient. Good risk management and ethical practice are usually compatible, but an unwarranted focus on malpractice risks can profoundly undermine the deliberations of HECs. Therefore, HECs should maintain close watch on the degree to which legal defensiveness, both justified and unjustified, influences their deliberations.

RECONCILING LAW AND ETHICS

Given the recognized dangers of overreliance on the law and risk management, it should be clear that our comments regarding the necessity and virtual inevitability of legal influence on HEC deliberations are descriptive, not normative. We are well of aware of the dangers of turning HECs into risk-management bodies and of mistaking law for ethics and ethics for law. Our only point is that conceptually, culturally, and practically, it will likely be impossible to sanitize HECs entirely from the leverage of the law. A more achievable and sensible goal would be to work toward understanding the appropriate role for law and legal involvement, participation, and integration in HEC deliberations.

In fact, how an HEC weighs these legal factors and integrates them into its discussions and recommendations can become an ethical issue in itself. Different HECs may develop different strategies to integrate legal considerations into ethical decision making. How should an HEC act in situations where legally correct practice is not necessarily synonymous with ethically correct practice? Should the law be bent or legal dangers ignored to provide more ethical care? Conversely, are there instances in which the most clinically and ethically appropriate action might be legitimately influenced by legal considerations? The answers to these questions will depend on the facts of the specific case and the various stakeholders. Patients, physicians, institutions, and HECs will have to decide together how they will weigh and balance patient needs, ethical duties, legal requirements, and risk. In doing so, however, it is important that they not mistake law for ethics, nor ethics for law.

Various measures might mitigate the danger that law will play too large a role in HEC discussions. For example, one potential approach might allow the ethics discussion to formulate and resolve the ethical and clinical questions involved in the case without a consideration of the legal issues involved. At that point, the legal issues can be addressed directly and, if there are conflicts between legal and ethical postures, then consider them at this juncture. In this way, the ethical and legal discussions are compartmentalized (albeit fictionally), and the distinction between the two can be maintained, and then reconciled (De Ville 1998). If, for example, the HEC is considering a problem or proposed policy that raises potential liability issues or risk issues, it may want to avoid ascribing undue weight to the risk of litigation (although a consideration of those risks is not irrelevant to the discussion). Faced with such a question, the HEC could: (1) evaluate the case; (2) make a clinically and ethically sound conclusion; (3) accurately identify the legal risk in the case; (4) evaluate the cost of the potential claim and its likelihood of occurring; and (5) consider the cost to the interests of the patient, physician, institution, and society of the potential defensive measure. Such an approach neither discounts legal risks nor raises them above other considerations, but it may allow HEC members to develop a responsible conception of what constitutes acceptable risk and remedies while keeping in mind the often independent goals of ethical decision making and risk management.

There are undoubtedly other ways to reconcile legitimately the overlapping influences of law and ethics. The most workable strategy will likely depend on the individual HEC's history, makeup, method of discussion, and interaction of members. Most thoughtful HEC members of good faith will find a way to deal with these complexities, as long as they are meaningfully aware of them.

THE PROBLEM WITH LAWYERS

Our discussion above outlines the potentially deleterious effect of law and legal discourse on HEC discussions but contends that law should not and probably cannot be banished from HEC deliberations. One of the reasons that the influence of law is felt so dramatically is that lawyers are frequent participants in, or members of, HECs (Buehler et al. 1989). From almost the advent of the HEC movement, some of the most perceptive commentators on the HEC phenomenon have attacked attorney participation in HEC discussions (Hastings Center 1987). Critics of attorney participation in ethics discussions voice a number of important warnings.

First, some attacks on attorney participation in HECs occasionally center on the claim that lawyers have not been trained to discuss moral issues related to medical care. Attorneys *are* trained primarily in law. But legal training does not necessarily render lawyers incapable of participating in discussions of the type occurring in HECs. There are clear analogies between the study of law and the study of moral philosophy. Law, like philosophy, places a premium on clear analysis, identification of key questions, cogent construction of arguments, and the refinement and critique of potential solutions. Both disciplines place a value on intellectual clarity and analytical rigor. These are skills that are helpful for ethical discussions in unraveling ethical questions and in weighing potential solutions. In addition, legal culture reflects a commitment to values highly relevant to bioethical discussions: equality, nondiscrimination, justice, individual rights, and autonomy. Thus, attorneys may possess, by nature of their training, many skills and habits of mind that might make them competent participants in moral discussions. Lawyers should not be automatically disqualified for membership by their training and avocation, and there are in fact good arguments for purposely including attorneys in HEC discussions. As noted earlier, in some instances, an accurate knowledge of the law and an appropriate evaluation of legal risks allow decision makers to pursue the path they deem most ethical, freeing clinicians' hands instead of tying them (De Ville and Hassler 2001; White 1991). Despite the growing degree of legal sophistication in HECs, many nonattorney members only know part of the law. Or, they may know the law technically and intellectually, yet misunderstand how it applies to the situation under consideration, that is, they know the law as written, not as applied. Competent and thoughtful attorneys can remedy this deficiency.

Second, perhaps the most common concern is that attorneys will place too great an emphasis on risk management or other legal aspects of the discussion to the exclusion of clinical, moral, or professional considerations. According to these commentators, a lawyer's aggressive legal opinion may shift the focus of the discussion from the ethical to the legal or end the discussion prematurely (Lowes 1992). As a result, ethical concerns may carry less weight in the analysis, which can have serious practical and ethical consequences for the medical staff, families, and patients. It is certainly true that attorneys should never mistake legal discourse for ethical discourse nor forget that the most appropriate legal course sometimes differs from the most appropriate ethical case. While in practice there are many attorneys who appear to have problems keeping this distinction in mind, there is no empirical evidence that lawyers, as a class, are intrinsically incapable of distinguishing between law and ethics. Connie Zuckerman's (1999) study of in-house counsel concluded that "it is unclear . . . whether hospital counsel really view patient care matters primarily through the same risk-averse lens or whether they can play a more reflective, thoughtful role within the facility, particularly regarding end-of-life care issues." Indeed, Zuckerman observed, many attorneys "appear to be comfortable responding to, and interpreting that law in a flexible, thoughtful manner in order to promote the wishes and interests of the patients and their families to the degree possible" (Zuckerman 1999). In fact, there are good reasons to suspect that thoughtful attorneys may be *less* likely to make this mistake than laypersons. Because they know the law better, they are more aware of its limitations. By professional disposition and habits of mind, attorneys may be better able to compartmentalize their professional roles, although they clearly do not always do so (De Ville and Hassler 2001). Finally, such fears, though often well founded, avoid the reality that medical ethicists, healthcare professionals, and other HEC members frequently discuss and reach conclusions about legal issues even if attorneys are not present, and these discussions may not always be well informed. A 1999 study of end-of-life care in hospitals found that "the focus of law was consistent" whether discussing the issues with institutional administrators, clinicians, or with hospital counsel (Zuckerman 1999). To make matters worse, there are empirical studies demonstrating that healthcare professionals have only a limited understanding of many key legal issues, yet nevertheless base clinical and ethical decisions on this limited understanding (McCrary et al. 1992). Therefore, the charge of excessive legalism can frequently be levied with equal concern at both lawyers and nonlawyers.

Third, critics of attorney participation in bioethical discussions frequently claim that institutional attorneys are faced with a species of conflict of interest, or, more properly stated, a conflict of commitment (Ross et al. 1993; Gottlieb 1991). That is, institutional counsel must act, on the one hand, as an advocate for the institution, and on the other hand, as a participant in a discussion with bioethical implications. These observers reason that attorneys' professional duty to advocate zealously for their clients will lead them to take an overly legalistic and conservative stance. Again, these fears and claims have some validity. Clearly, attorneys sometimes favor the safest, most conservative legal position, especially if that is what their client desires. However, that is not always what the client desires, especially in the healthcare delivery setting. Zealous representation of clients need not be—and usually is not—a single-minded goal, especially in the healthcare field and especially when asked to serve in a dual role by the client, like serving on or advising an HEC. The client may want the attorney to find a *safe* legal stance consistent with other organizational goals, not necessarily the *safest*. Therefore, it is important to find out exactly what the client (institutional or otherwise) wants the attorney's role to be in the particular case at hand and cases like it. The American Bar Association (ABA) Model Rules of Professional Conduct and the ABA Model Code make it clear that attorneys may consider other issues than the purely legal: "In rendering advice, an attorney may refer not only to law but to other considerations such as moral, economic, social and political factors that may be relevant to the client's situation." Quite simply, attorneys are not limited by their profession to the unitary goal of risk management. Again, the common complaint that attorneys are excessively risk averse misses the important point that many nonlawyers involved in medical ethical discussions, too, have nearly equal motivation to be risk averse and to protect the institution and perhaps themselves (De Ville and Hassler 2001; White 1991; Kapp and Lo 1986).

Despite these comments that attorneys are not irretrievably biased or bound by their professional training, there is merit to the claim that an attorney's professional tendencies, intellectual background, and institutional role may sometimes be incongruent with what is the most ethical decision. It is important that individuals who serve on and consult HECs realize that the lawyer with whom they deal may wear two hats for the purpose of ethical and legal discussions. *Disclosure* is a time-honored prophylactic measure when conflicts of interest or commitment, or their appearance, is involved. It may be appropriate in the contexts of HECs too. Disclosure should include a clear articulation of when the attorney is speaking as a legal advocate and when the attorney is speaking as a participant in an ethical discussion. If an attorney cannot reconcile his or her dual roles in bioethical discussions, then perhaps this is not the correct work for him or her and recusal becomes appropriate. Attorneys involved with HECs might benefit from the above proposed strategy that suggests allowing the ethics discussion to formulate and resolve the ethical and clinical issues with the case without consideration of the legal issues involved. At that point, if legal issues remain, they can be addressed openly and reconciled. This compartmentalization might mitigate the potentially distracting effect of legal concerns (De Ville and Hassler 2001). As Judith Wilson Ross advises, a lawyer who serves on an HEC should have the same qualities required of other members, namely, "an openness to discussion, a willingness to participate, the ability to listen to others, the ability to focus on the goals and charge of the HEC, and an interest in the ethical aspects of health care." If the lawyer does not have these qualities, the HEC "would likely be better off without one as a member" (Ross et al. 1993).

CONCLUSION

Given the intellectual and institutional history of bioethics and HECs, it is not surprising that law continues to influence HECs and to shape HEC discussions of substantive issues. In addition, legal considerations and legal habits of mind will likely continue to influence HECs because the issues committees regularly face necessarily raise both legal and ethical questions, and because HEC members are drawn from a culture in which, rightly or wrongly, law is equated with rights, justice, and morality. To paraphrase Marshall Kapp, "in specific cases law and ethics may be synonymous, distinct, at odds, complementary, or overlapping," but that influence is always there (Kapp 1999). It would be unrealistic to expect that the law's influence could be, or should be, exiled from the hearts and minds of HEC members, their discourse, and their deliberations. If courts give more explicit weight to the conclusions of HECs, it will become even more difficult to suggest realistically that the influence of law can or should be banned from these deliberations. It will loom even larger and provide a more potent part of the subtext of every HEC discussion. The most for which one can hope is a fuller and more sophisticated conception and integration of law's role in and influence on HEC deliberations.

FOR FURTHER REFLECTION

1. How has the law historically shaped and informed the evolution of HECs?
2. In what ways do legal considerations of bioethics issues benefit HECs? How do such perspectives limit HECs?
3. Are there decisional contexts within the practice of medicine that should exclude legal analyses? If so, what is the specific context and the decisional framework HECs should follow?

4. Hypothetical: an HEC attorney-member consistently eschews moral complexities of bioethics issues before HEC, consistently warns HEC that it fails to grasp fully the practical risks with some of its decisions, and makes it clear her interests are those of the institution and not the physician or patient. How would you would talk with the attorney-member concerning her perspectives?

WORKS CITED

Annas, G. J. 1991. Ethics committees: From ethical comfort to ethical cover. *Hastings Center Report* 21 (3): 18–21.

———. 1993. *Standard of care: The law of American bioethics*. New York and Oxford: Oxford University Press.

Balkin, J. 1986. The crystalline structure of legal thought. *Rutgers Law Review* 39:1–77.

Brody, H. 1989. Transparency: Informed consent in primary care. *Hastings Center Report* 19 (5): 5–9.

Buehler, D. A., R. M. DiVita, and J. J. Yium. 1989. Hospital ethics committees: The hospital attorney's role. *HEC Forum* 1 (4): 183–94.

Capron, A. M. 1999. What contributions have social science and the law made to the development of policy on bioethics? *Daedalus* 128 (4): 295–325.

Cranford, R. E., and A. E. Doudera. 1984. Institutional ethics committees and health care decision making. *Law, Medicine, & Ethics* 12 (1): 13–19.

De Ville, K. A. 1994. What does the law say?: Law, ethics, and medical decision making. *Western Journal of Medicine* 160 (5): 478–80.

———. 1998. Act first and look up the law afterward? Medical malpractice and the ethics of defensive practice. *Theoretical Medicine and Bioethics* 19 (6): 569–89.

De Ville, K. A, and G. Hassler. 2001. Law and health care ethics committees: Uneasy but inevitable bedfellows. *HEC Forum* 13 (1): 13–31.

Dworkin, R. B. 1996. *Limits: The role of law in bioethics decision making*.

Flamm, A. L. 2000. Texas takes on medical futility. *ASBH Exchange*. http://www.asbh .org/exchange/2000/w00flamm.htm (accessed January 8, 2005).

Fleetwood, J., R. M. Arnold, and R. J. Baron. 1989. Giving answers or raising questions? The problematic role of institutional ethics committees. *Journal of Medical Ethics* 15 (3): 137–42.

Gottlieb, L. E. 1991. Point and counterpoint: Should an institution's risk manager/ lawyer serve as HEC members? No. *HEC Forum* 3 (2): 91–93.

Hart, H. L. A. 1961. *The concept of law*. New York: Oxford University Press.

Hastings Center. 1987. *Guidelines on the termination of life sustaining treatment and the care for the dying*. New York: Hastings Center.

Hoffman, D. E. 1991. Hospital ethics committees and the law: Regulating ethics committees in health care institutions. *Maryland Law Review* 50:746–97.

Holmes, O. W. 1897. The path of the law. *Harvard Law Review* 10:457–58.

Kapp, M. B. 1999. *Our hands are tied: Legal tensions and medical ethics*. Westport, CT: Auburn House.

Kapp, M. B, and B. Lo. 1986. Legal perceptions and medical decision making. *The Milbank Quarterly* 64 (Supp. 2): 163–201.

Lowes, R. L. 1992. How and ethics panel can—and can't—help you. *Medical Economics* 69: 166–68, 173, 176–83.

McCrary, S. V., J. W. Swanson, H. S. Perkins, and W. J. Winslade. 1992. Treatment decisions for terminally ill patients: Physicians' legal defensiveness and knowledge of medical law. *Law, Medicine, and Healthcare* 20:364–76.

Murphy, J. F., and J. L. Coleman. 1990. *Philosophy of law: An introduction to jurisprudence.* Boulder, San Francisco, and London: Westview Press.

Povar, G. 1991. Hospital ethics committees and the law: Evaluating ethics committees: What do we mean by success? *Maryland Law Review* 50:904–19.

Powell, L. T. 1998. Hospital ethics committees and the future of health care decision making. *Hospital Material Management Quarterly* 20 (1): 82–90.

President's Commission for the Study of Ethical Problems in Medicine and Biomedical Research. 1983. *Deciding to forego life-sustaining treatment: Ethical, medical, and legal issues in treatment decisions.* Washington, DC: U.S. Government Printing Office.

Quinlan. 1976. *In re Quinlan.* 70 N. J. 10, 355 A.2d 647 (1976).

Ross, J. W. 1996. Editor's introduction. *HEC Forum* 8 (6): 327–29.

Ross, J. W., J. W. Glaser, D. Rasinski-Gregory, J. M. Gibson, and C. Bayley. 1993. *Health care ethics committees: The next generation.* American Hospital Association.

Saikewicz. 1977. *Superintendent of Belchertown State School v. Saikewicz.* 372 Mass. 728, 370 N.E. 2d 417 (1977).

Scott, C. 2000. Why law pervades medicine: An essay on ethics in health care. *Notre Dame Journal of Law, Ethics & Public Policy* 14:245–302.

Spring. 1980. *In re Spring.* 380 Mass. 629, 405 N.E. 2d 115 (1980).

Torres. 1984. *In re Torres.* 357 N.W. 2d 332 (Minn. 1984).

White, B. 1991. Point and counterpoint: Should an institution's risk manager/lawyer serve as HEC members? Yes. *HEC Forum* 3 (2): 87–89.

Wilson, R. F. 1998. Hospital ethics as a forum of last resort: An idea whose time has not yet come. *North Carolina Law Review* 76:353–406.

Wolf, S. M. 1991. Hospital ethics committees and the law: Ethics committees and due process: Nesting rights in a community of caring. *Maryland Law Review* 50:798–858.

Zuckerman, C. 1999. *End-of-life care and hospital legal counsel: Current involvement and opportunities for the future.* New York: Milbank Memorial Fund.

15

A Management Guide for the Committee

Eugene J. Kuc

KEY POINTS

1. Group dynamics are present whenever two or more people gather to perform a task. Being attentive to these processes and identifying destructive processes early may help the group be more successful and save the members much time and strife.
2. This chapter will review work and nonwork dynamics, definition of roles and tasks, and stages of group development. The material will help the reader be better prepared for work on a hospital ethics committee (HEC), as examples (including interventions) pertinent to this work are included.

The previous chapters have discussed components of the work performed by an HEC with attention to technical knowledge and specialized skills. And yet, little attention has been paid to working within the and as a committee itself. Almost every committee member can recall meetings during which it seemed as if no work was accomplished or that the discussion had nothing to do with the formal charge of the committee. She or he may also recall times when the committee seemed to be caught in a wave of sentiment that unwittingly stifled dissent or ignored other, maybe even more rational, forces. How do we explain this? More important, how might we respond when we find ourselves in these situations? Better yet, how can we avoid these situations altogether? This chapter is intended to serve as a committee management guide in light of just these aspects of group dynamics.

COMMITTEES AS GROUPS:
FOCUSING ON THE TASK AT HAND

The first issue to consider when discussing groups is how best to define a group. Rice (1963; Miller and Rice 1967) defines a group as individuals working on a "primary task." In turn, Rice defines a "primary task" as that task which the group needs to perform in order to survive. Examples are numerous from industry to education—for example, the Ford Motor Company is organized to produce automobiles (primary task), or a patient-care group works on patient-care issues in a hospital (primary task). In this way, the task defines the group. While groups may have secondary tasks such as charitable endeavors, training activities, and so on, the primary task is that which the group must perform in order to continue to exist as the group it purports to be. Too much attention to secondary tasks often leads to the demise of the group. In this light, then, an HEC exists as a group in order to fulfill the mission given it by the institution. Though the primary task may vary mildly from institution to institution, most HECs are primarily charged with the task of providing consultation to patients, family, and staff in ethically complex medical care. Secondary tasks often include activities such as education and training, policy review, or consultation; however, in many situations, if the HEC stops responding effectively to the requests for consults, the committee will become impotent or simply will not survive.[1]

A useful distinction has been made by Bion (1961) in characterizing two types of groups: "work groups" and "basic assumption groups." A work group exists when a group is focused on its primary task. On the other hand, when a group loses its focus on the primary or secondary tasks, Bion describes the group as a basic assumption group, of which there are three types: basic assumption dependence, basic assumption pairing, and basic assumption fight-flight. Groups engaged in basic assumption processes act as if they are doing work, but in fact they are avoiding real work.

According to Bion, basic assumption dependence occurs when a group acts as if it cannot initiate work until a leader emerges to guide them; the group colludes to await a leader to rescue them. Often, such groups will discuss and sometimes outright fantasize about a competent person coming to lead. This type of group behavior can result in otherwise-competent individuals becoming impotent as they defer decisions until a savior arrives. If a group member takes on the role of the leader, a period of idealization and ecstasy often follows, with the group finding the leader nearly infallible; however, soon thereafter the pendulum swings, and the leader is dismissed as incompetent, resulting in the need to search for a new leader. Often the new leader is dismissed immediately. Much debate occurs within the group as to the qualities of this sought-after savior, who might be a potential candidate, and so forth; in the meantime, no work takes place because it is precisely the avoidance of work through this preoccupation with a fantasized future leader that is the unconscious goal of the group. The manifestation of this process during the work of an HEC could involve dialogue of how an ideally trained leader could deal with a particularly difficult situation and identify the appropriate ethical principles by which the consultation should be guided—yet no such leader comes forward or is available, and the group is left longing and searching—a search that may continue indefinitely. Beyond a preoccupation with leadership, basic assumption dependence can involve a conscious, or unconscious, preoccupation in the group with furthering a particular ideology, worrying about financial stability and ability, as well as political (or other seemingly fundamental) concerns. This preoccupation comes at the expense of balanced discussions, and thus, such a mistargeted focus and dependence on guiding forces can be quite destructive to the primary task of the HEC.

Basic assumption pairing, as another version of basic assumption groups, is characterized as a group process where two group members pair off and essentially discuss the goals for leadership and direction of the group. While neither of the members themselves will take on the leadership role, the actions of these two individuals are somehow intended to give birth to this leader or directing principle. The rest of the group becomes complicit in encouraging the pair to continue working toward the identification of this new leader or direction, which perpetuates the hope that a messiah or messianic principle will rescue the group. Of course, an actual messiah is not desired, as that would mean the group would have to return to the primary work task. This can be seen, for example, in an HEC that encourages two members to prolong a debate about the merits of different theoretical approaches, while the HEC itself stands at an impasse. The rest of the committee will encourage the two members to continue debate, seemingly hoping that they reach a resolution that would magically resolve the situation, but in actuality, the unspoken goal becomes one of prolonging this debate as much as possible in order to avoid work.

Last, basic assumption fight-flight is another way in which real work can be avoided by investing energy in battling or avoiding an enemy. Under basic assumption fight-flight, some individual, group, ideology, or other similar "villain" is seen as a threat to the group, and rather than focusing on creating a legitimate product through legitimate work, the group focuses on various aspects of the "enemy"— how to revile and defeat or avoid it. Much energy is devoted to defining and vilifying the enemy, and all the while, no progress is made toward group work on its primary task. An example of this process is when a particular person, department, ideology, organization, and so forth is seen as a challenge or adversary to which the group decides it needs to respond. For an HEC, this may manifest with a group consensus that persons in a particular department are not sympathetic to the committee's efforts, to good medical care generally, or to a particular patient or patient's needs. This person or department is then judged as bad or incompetent, and the HEC then fantasizes about the various ways by which the people in this department could be changed; while this fantasizing is occurring, the HEC neglects the true work: the requested consultation.

While no one of these basic assumptions will necessarily prevail in every HEC, *every* group will find itself at various times engaged in one or more of the basic assumptions for various lengths of time, and every group member is responsible as an equal participant— whether vocal or not. The response inevitably involves redirecting back to the legitimate official primary task of the group; often, acknowledging the group's ambivalence about engaging in the work helps facilitate this redirection. Typically, the emotional tone of a group involved in a basic assumption process is that of anxiety, while the emotional state of a work group is devoid of this anxiety.

GROUP STRUCTURE: LEADERS AND MEMBERS

There are many different kinds of legitimate organizational structures that can lead to successful work groups ("organizational structure," here, refers to models that define authority, chain of command, and so forth). Strict and formal hierarchical systems can be just as effective as less-formal structures, and it is beyond the scope of this brief chapter to comment on the nuances of working within the various systems. However, what is useful to consider are various roles within the group, since many roles are present regardless of how the organization is structured. In particular, two main roles to consider are those of group leader and group member.

When considering aspects of leadership, three concepts are often involved: authority, leadership, and power. *Authority* involves officially recognized expertise and responsibility that arises from a formal appointment process such as an election, accreditation, or appointment. Persons who hold positions of authority are accountable for performing specific duties—for example, department chairs managing the finances of their department. *Leadership* does not involve any formal designation of responsibility, but rather an informal process is involved: one or more people identify an individual as having particular skills and choose to follow that person's lead. These individuals are often seen as the experts in the department or the champions of a particular cause, though they may not have any official title or recognition. *Power* involves neither formal nor informal responsibility, nor does it involve expertise or influence. Rather, power involves an ability to do something through physical or phychological force. For example, a person walking into a bank may have no authority or leadership role, but the moment the individual pulls out a gun and makes demands, this person is in a position of power and will affect a group's behavior. Further, individuals who control finances, data sets, potentially embarrassing personal information, and so on may be seen as operating from a position of power rather than authority or leadership. Individuals can hold positions involving all three components at the same time, can have combinations of two, or may flow through various roles while working in a group. For purposes of this discussion, the word "leader" will be used in the normatively positive sense that assumes a benevolent and appropriate use of all three aspects described above.

With that said, the leader's main responsibility is to help keep the group focused on the appropriate primary and secondary tasks and to secure the resources necessary for the group to perform this work. The leader often splits time focusing on the work within the group while also being attentive to outside forces and resources that may impact the group; this is also known as managing boundaries. The leader of an HEC would be responsible for, among other things, securing appropriate resources for the committee—meeting place, administrative support, effective communication methods, access to specialized bodies of knowledge, and so on. The committee leader dialogues and negotiates with leaders of other departments and superiors to assure the effective functioning of the group. The leader can and often does delegate many of these tasks.

Though not unique to an HEC, the HEC leader must also be careful to keep dialogue open, promoting participation of members. Committee work in ethics, and especially ethics consultation, has as its greatest resource the expertise of the members. The leader would be expected to manage this resource by inviting all members of the HEC to be included in the discussion, even if theirs is a dissenting voice against a critical mass rallying around a particular position. This is no easy task at times, but good leadership in an HEC recognizes that the outcome of an HEC ethics deliberation aims at the best possible solution for the situation, not just for any particular point of view (whether that be institutional, physician, or patient interests).

As such, the role of members is to use their specific expertise and skills to further work toward the primary task, according to the responsibilities placed on the member. For example, it would be expected of physician members of the HEC to contribute medical knowledge pertinent to the patient being discussed, and if there is no physician member, one could rightly question the ability of the HEC to achieve its task of a complete ethics consultation in a medical setting. Presence or absence of representatives from legal, religious, administrative, financial, ethics, psychological, and other disciplines will clearly influence the nature of the discussion and thus the consultation results of the committee (see chapter 1 herein).

An important and often unconscious role members also take on is that of processing and containing emotions. These emotions, and the beliefs associated with them, that individual group members tend to adopt are known as valences. Group members may have a tendency to be the "voice of reason" or to be leader or even victim or any of a myriad of possible valences. An awareness of one's own valences and the valences of others, while encouraging the sharing of data from all perspectives, is important to the group process and the work. If one group member tends to take on the victim's valence, for example, and remains silent during a consultation in which the patient may be seen in the position of victim, a full appreciation of this process with discussion of possible interventions to address this dynamic could be missed, leading to a suboptimal consultation. Indeed, if there is an uncomfortable silence within the group, one would suspect that work is not being done and that a basic assumption is present (often a member may be or seem to be exerting power leading to oppression, leading to the submissive silence). Thus, looking for the etiology of the oppression and redirecting to work is important to get the group back on track. While a leader should be keenly aware of such dynamics in the group, all members have an equal responsibility to make the group's efforts effective.

GROUP DEVELOPMENT

Groups are dynamic, and the forces that influence a group are fluid and shifting. The discussion thus far is pertinent to any stage of group development. However, as dynamic, groups are organic and developing. Thus, attention to generally accepted stages of group development may lessen the anxiety associated with working in a group and participating in the group process. While the reader is cautioned against adopting an overly simplistic literal interpretation of the group development process as groups do not at all need to achieve all the stages or progress in any sequential manner, planning for each of these stages may prove useful. One widely accepted model of group development was put forth by Tuckman (1965; Tuckman and Jensen 1977), who described the evolution of a group involving five stages: forming, storming, norming, performing, and adjourning.

Forming is defined as the stage when a group first comes together and starts to develop common definitions, assign roles, and reach agreement on the primary task. *Storming* often follows when these agreed-upon definitions, roles, and tasks are challenged and there is resistance to full consensus and engagement. Negotiation then follows during the *norming* stage, when cohesiveness of the group develops to a near-operational level and roles and other definitions evolve in order to meet consensus. *Performing* follows, which is the stage during which the work toward the primary task is at its most efficient. Definitions and roles adapt and become more flexible to accommodate needs in order to continue effectively achieving the task. *Adjourning*, then, is when the primary task is completed and there is no further need for the group; at this stage, group members often have feelings of sadness and anxiety as well as nostalgia and reflection on the work and shared experiences. This model can be applied to a single meeting of a group or to a series of meetings; an HEC can be seen as going through all of these stages during one meeting, or while working over several meetings on a particular consultation, or under the tenure of a particular administration or chair.

Awareness of these dynamics and stages can help the group member navigate specific processes by being able to identify when the group has lost its focus on the primary (or legitimate secondary) tasks and redirecting the group back to the appropriate tasks, maintaining appropriate boundaries of roles and tasks, and managing the emotions in the group.

CONCLUSION

Work in groups is influenced by known group processes, and the work of an HEC is no exception. Awareness of the basic principles of group dynamics can assist the HEC member in responding to these forces as they manifest themselves and help redirect the HEC to its primary task. Many conceptual models exist to organize thinking about these issues, and in this chapter, several classic theories about factors that influence the activity in a group were presented. The reader is encouraged to explore additional texts on this topic and to consider consultation from organizational experts if group dynamics seem to be adversely affecting or perhaps even preventing the effective functioning of the HEC.

FOR FURTHER REFLECTION

1. The reader is challenged to reflect on the exact nature of the primary task of his or her HEC and to see if there is agreement among the other members.
2. The reader is challenged to explore if the nature of his or her work actually furthers the primary task of the HEC.
3. Using the basic tools with which one can identify the group process occurring in an HEC, the reader is encouraged to reflect on his or her own role in perpetuating basic assumption processes, and further, he or she is encouraged to attempt redi-

rection of those processes to legitimate primary and secondary tasks.

4. The reader is encouraged to reflect on his or her own personal valences.

NOTE

1. A classic movie often used by teachers of group dynamics is the original 1957 version of *Twelve Angry Men* starring Peter Fonda as a member of a jury deliberating a verdict on a capital murder trial. Many other agendas creep into the action, to which members of the jury artfully respond, but it is only the arrival at a verdict that is legitimate work, the primary task.

WORKS CITED

Bion, W. R. 1961. *Experiences in groups.* London: Tavistock Publications.

Rice, A. K. 1963. *The enterprise and its environment.* London: Tavistock Publications.

Miller, E. J., and A. K. Rice. 1967. *Systems of organization: Task and sentient systems and their boundary control.* London: Tavistock Publications.

Tuckman, B. W. 1965. Developmental sequence in small groups. *Psychological Bulletin* 63:384–99.

Tuckman, B. W., and M. A. Jensen. 1977. Stages of small-group development revisited. *Group & Organization Studies* 2: 419–27.

Further Resources

The literature on biomedical ethics is growing rapidly, and there is no way to be comprehensive. The following, then, are offered as next steps in the educational process for HEC members, and should be used in conjunction with other works cited at the end of chapters herein.

I. BOOKS

American Hospital Association. 1994. *Values in conflict: Resolving ethical issues in health care.* 2nd ed. Chicago: American Hospital Association.

American Society for Bioethics and Humanities, *Core Competencies for Ethics Consultations* (1998). The product of a multisociety taskforce (SHHV/SBC) that provides guidance about concepts and skills that ground ethics consultation.

Beauchamp T, Childress J, *The Principles of Biomedical Ethics*, 5th ed. (Oxford University Press, 2001). A theoretically rigorous discussion of the basic principles of medical ethics, but it can be rough going for the impatient beginner or the clinician with an immediate problem to solve.

Fry ST, Veatch RM, *Case Studies in Nursing Ethics*, 3rd ed. (Jones and Bartlett, 2006). Provides insight for ethical issues experienced in nursing practice.

Glannon W, *Biomedical Ethics* (Oxford Univ. Press, 2004). A straightforward, short volume concerning primary concepts and issues in medical ethics.

Jonsen, Siegler, Winslade, *Clinical Ethics*, 5th ed. (McGraw-Hill, 2002). Written for clinicians, it gives a balanced overview of medical ethics and provides some recommendations on specific issues. Short on theoretical discussions.

Kuczewski MG, Pinkus RLB, *An Ethics Casebook for Hospitals* (Georgetown UP, 1999). Provides cases and analyses of everyday situations that hospital healthcare professionals might encounter.

Kushner TK, Thomasma DC, *Ward Ethics* (Cambridge UP, 2001). Discusses ethical issues from the perspective of medical students and other professionals in training.

Pence G, *Classic Cases in Medical Ethics*, 4th ed. (McGraw-Hill, 2004). A readable and readily accessible introduction to bioethics through landmark cases.

Post LF, Blustein J, Dubler NN, *Handbook for Health Care Ethics Committees* (Johns Hopkins, 2006). A resource targeted to the issues that HECs face.

Reich W (ed.), *The Encyclopedia of Bioethics*, 1st ed. (Macmillan, 1989), 2nd ed. (Macmillan, 1995), and Post, S (ed.), 3rd ed. (Macmillan, 2003). The only comprehensive, general resource in bioethics.

Ross, JW, JW Glaser, D Rasinski-Gregory, JM Gibson, and C Bayler. 1993. *Health care ethics committees: The next generation.* Chicago: Jossey-Bass AHA Press.

II. PERIODICALS

Selected journals that either focus on or often have articles on bioethics and medical humanities—there are others, however, so keep searching: PubMed— http://www.ncbi.nlm.nih.gov/entrez/query.fcgi.

American Journal of Bioethics
Bioethics
Cambridge Quarterly of Health Care Ethics
Ethics & Medicine
Hastings Center Report
HEC (Healthcare Ethics Committee) Forum
Journal of Clinical Ethics
Journal of Law, Medicine & Ethics
Journal of Medical Ethics
Kennedy Institute of Ethics Journal
Theoretical Medicine and Bioethics

III. WEBSITES

Bioethics Resources on the Web: National Institutes of Health
   http://www.nih.gov/sigs/bioethics/. This website contains a broad collage of annotated Web links, and while the list is comprehensive, it is not totally inclusive. The listed resources provide background information and various positions on issues in bioethics.

Bioethics.net
   http://bioethics.net. Contains news and information related to bioethical issues and is associated with the *American Journal of Bioethics*, Albany Medical College, University of Pennsylvania, and Stanford University.

Pediatric Ethics Consortium
   http://www.pediatricethics.org. Contains information, links, and archived resources in pediatric ethics.

Virtual Mentor
> http://www.ama-assn.org/ama/pub/category/3040.html. The American Medical Association's ethics and humanities website, published as an online periodical with articles and case studies.

IV. VIDEOS

Code Gray (Fanlight Productions, 47 Halifax Street, Boston, MA 02130, $245.00). Four vignettes that illustrate the principles of beneficence, autonomy, justice, and fidelity. Features nurses discussing application of the principles to the cases.

Deception (Institute for the Study of Applied and Professional Ethics, Dartmouth College, Hanover, NH 03755). A doctor and nurse, and ultimately an ethics committee, deliberate about telling a woman whose husband has just died that he gave her syphilis.

Dax's Case (Choice in Dying, 200 Varick Street, New York, NY 10014). Dax Cowart was severely burned and was treated for months over his repeated requests to be discharged. Interviews with everyone involved in the case. Also on CD-ROM is "A Right To Die? The Dax Cowart Case" (Routledge), interactive ethics education software.

Index

About the Contributors

Dyrleif Bjarnadottir, MA, MSBioethics, is a research fellow at the Alden March Bioethics Institute in Albany, New York, and is currently working on her PhD dissertation in reproductive ethics. Her most recent research projects include issues of newborn screening and states' responsibilities, the obligations of parents to their children, and the cultural variance in the significance of parental autonomy in treatment decisions for neonates.

Mark J. Bliton, PhD, is an associate professor of medical ethics and of obstetrics and gynecology in the Vanderbilt University School of Medicine as well as an associate professor of philosophy in Vanderbilt's College of Arts & Sciences. He served (1994–2007) as chief of Vanderbilt University Medical Center's Clinical Ethics Consultation Service and is the area director for medical humanities within the medical school's innovative Emphasis Program. His areas of academic interest include the values expressed in innovative maternal-fetal surgical interventions, which were the focus of "Parental Voices in Maternal-Fetal Surgery," featured in the recent volume of *Clinical Obstetrics and Gynecology* (2005) that he coedited with Larry R. Churchill. Other areas of clinical and academic interest include the complexity of ethics in the neonatal intensive care setting and moral experience in the context of patient care.

Michael Boylan, PhD, is professor of philosophy and chair of philosophy at Marymount University. He is the author of seventeen books and over eighty articles covering ethics, philosophy of science, and philosophy in literature. His most recent books include *A Just Society* (2004), *Basic Ethics* (2000), *Genetic Engineering: Science and Ethics on the New Frontier* (2002, with Kevin E. Brown), *Ethics across the Curriculum: A Practice-Based Approach* (2003, with

James A. Donahue), and *Public Health Policy and Ethics* (ed. 2004). He has been invited to lecture in eight countries and on three continents.

Kenneth A. De Ville, PhD, JD, is professor at Brody School of Medicine in Greenville, North Carolina. His research interests include legal medicine, bioethics, and the history of medical jurisprudence. De Ville is the author of *Medical Malpractice in Nineteenth-Century America: Origins and Legacy* (1990) and coeditor of *Physician Assisted Suicide: What Are the Issues?* (2002). He has authored numerous articles and book chapters including peer-reviewed publications in journals such as: *The Journal of Medicine and Philosophy; Journal of Health Care Compliance; Clinics in Obstetrics and Gynecology; Law, Medicine, and Ethics; Theoretical Medicine and Bioethics; The Journal of Clinical Ethics; American Journal of Bioethics; The Historian; Pediatrics; Trends in Health Care, Law, and Ethics; Current Surgery; HEC Forum; Cambridge Quarterly of Healthcare Ethics; The International Journal of Technology Assessment in Health Care; The Missouri Law Review; American Journal of Public Health; Mount Sinai Medical Journal; Seminars in Pediatric Surgery; Academic Medicine; Defense Counsel Journal; Accountability in Research;* and *The Journal of Legal Medicine.* De Ville has served on numerous ethics review committees and panels, is a member of the North Carolina Bar, and serves as "Of Counsel" to two North Carolina health-law firms.

Stuart G. Finder, PhD, is director of the Center for Healthcare Ethics and chief of bioethics at Cedars-Sinai Medical Center in Los Angeles, California. Prior to this appointment, he served as an assistant professor and clinical ethics consultant for Vanderbilt University Medical Center (VUMC), cochair of VUMC's Ethics Committee, and the senior associate director of VUMC's Center for Biomedical Ethics and Society. He also served for six years (2001–2007) on the American Society of Bioethics and Humanities' Task Force on Clinical Ethics, where he played a central role in the development of the ASBH's "Improving Competence in Clinical Ethics Consultation: A Learner's Guide." His main areas of academic interest include the ethical considerations associated with clinical ethics consultation practice and the moral features of clinical contexts more generally.

Richard E. Grant, MD, is the Edgar B. Jackson, MD, Chair for Clinical Excellence and Diversity and professor of orthopedics, total joint replacement, and adult reconstruction at Case Western Reserve University and University Hospitals. He is former president of the American Board of Orthopedic Surgeons. In ethics, he has worked on issues of professionalism and the theory of deserts. Grant and Michael Boylan have teamed up on articles ranging from assessing diversity and medical excellence to end-of-life care to social/medical assessments of our healthcare delivery system.

Chris Hackler, PhD, is professor and director of the Division of Medical Humanities of the College of Medicine, University of Arkansas for Medical Sciences, and Inaugural Professor in the University of Arkansas's Clinton School of Public Service. He received a PhD in philosophy from the University of North Carolina and has held awards from the Woodrow Wilson Foundation, the Fulbright Commission, and the National Endowment for the Humanities. Dr. Hackler was a founding member of his own hospital's ethics committee twenty years ago and has helped establish HECs in several other institutions. He has published primarily on end-of-life issues and on heath-care policy.

Gregory L. Hassler, JD, PhD, has served, since 1990, East Carolina University as chief legal counsel of its Brody School of Medicine and as associate university attorney of its Health Sciences Division, which includes the Schools of Nursing and Allied Health Sciences. He holds JD and PhD degrees from Emory University and maintains licenses in North Carolina and Georgia.

D. Micah Hester, PhD, is assistant professor of medical humanities and pediatrics at the University of Arkansas for Medical Sciences and clinical ethicist at Arkansas Children's Hospital. He has authored or edited seven books, including *Community as Healing* (2001) with Rowman & Littlefield, and numerous journal articles and commentaries. His scholarly interests have focused on professional-patient relationships, end-of-life care, and transplant issues. Dr. Hester has long been concerned with ethics education and spends time developing course work for medical students, residents, attending physicians, nurses, social workers, and other healthcare professionals. His current and previous service on several HECs and IRBs inspired him to develop the present volume.

Lynn A. Jansen, PhD, is an associate research professor in the Department of Medicine and the assistant director of The Bioethics Institute at New York Medical College. She is also senior medical ethicist at St. Vincent's Manhattan.

Nancy S. Jecker, PhD, is professor of medical ethics at the University of Washington School of Medicine, Department of Medical History and Ethics. She is adjunct professor at the University of Washington School of Law and Department of Philosophy. Her research interests include ethical theory, justice and health care, and ethical decisions to withhold and withdraw medical treatment. Dr. Jecker is editor (with Albert Jonsen and Robert Pearlman) of the forthcoming book, *Bioethics: An Introduction to the History, Methods, and Practice*, 2nd edition (2007). She is the author (with Lawrence

Schneiderman) of *Wrong Medicine: Doctors, Patients, and Futile Treatment* (1995). Dr. Jecker has authored over one hundred articles and chapters on ethics and health care. Her articles have appeared in *The Journal of the American Medical Association, The Hastings Center Report, Annals of Internal Medicine, The Journal of Medicine and Philosophy*, and other publications.

Kathy Kinlaw, MDiv, is acting director of the Emory University Center for Ethics and director of the center's program in health-sciences ethics. She serves as bioethics associate in pediatrics, Emory School of Medicine, and executive director of the Health Care Ethics Consortium of Georgia. Since 1994, she has codirected the School of Medicine's required third-year course on clinical ethics. Her publications and scholarly interests are primarily in the areas of palliative and end-of-life care, ethics and medical education, perinatal and neonatal ethics, the work of ethics committees, and public health ethics. Kathy serves as a member of the CDC's Ethics Committee to the Advisory Council to the Director and is on the Georgia Composite Board of Medical Examiners. Prior to joining the Center for Ethics in 1990, Kathy completed a fellowship in perinatal ethics at the Department of Pediatrics, Emory School of Medicine. She obtained her Master of Divinity degree from Emory's Candler School of Theology, where she was a Woodruff Scholar. Kathy served as an intern at the Office of Bioethics at the National Institutes of Health and participated in the Washington Semester in Theology and Public Policy at Wesley Theological Seminary in Washington, DC.

Tracy K. Koogler, MD, is an associate professor of pediatrics in Pediatric Critical Care at the University of Chicago. She is also on faculty at the MacLean Center for Clinical Medical Ethics and is the codirector of the ethics consultation service. Her research interests are in the physician-patient-family relationship in pediatrics, pediatric palliative care, and organ donation.

Eugene J. Kuc, MD, is an associate professor in the Department of Psychiatry and Behavioral Sciences at the University of Arkansas for Medical Sciences and a staff physician at the Central Arkansas Veterans Healthcare System. He is involved both locally and internationally with quality improvement and hospital accreditation initiatives. Clinical areas of expertise include the treatment of trauma and personality disorders. He is course director for the course on group dynamics for residents in psychiatry at UAMS. He received postgraduate and fellowship training at the University of Illinois at Chicago; his fellowship was in organizational and administrative psychiatry.

Timothy F. Murphy, PhD, holds a doctorate in philosophy from Boston College and is professor of philosophy in the biomedical sciences at the

University of Illinois College of Medicine at Chicago. He conducts research and teaches primarily in the areas of genetics and ethics, assisted reproductive technologies, medicine and sexuality, and research ethics. He is the author or editor of eight books, including most recently *Case Studies in Biomedical Research Ethics* (2004). With grant support from the Department of Defense, in 1991, he convened one of the first national conferences dealing with the ethics of the Human Genome Project. He has also received grant support from the National Institutes of Health for work related to the ethical, legal, and social implications of research. He convened two national conferences during that grant: "Research Ethics: Confronting Challenges in the Next Millennium" (1999) and "Research Ethics at the Frontiers of Medicine" (2001). Professor Murphy is a member of the ethics committees of the American College of Surgeons Oncology Group and the American Academy of Pain Medicine. He has also been a visiting scholar at the Institute for Ethics of the American Medical Association in Chicago.

David T. Ozar, PhD, is professor and codirector of graduate studies in healthcare ethics, Department of Philosophy, Loyola University Chicago. He has also taught in Loyola's schools of medicine, nursing, business, law, education, social work, and dentistry. He served as director of Loyola's Center for Ethics and Social Justice (1993–2006). He has taught at Loyola since 1972. In addition to his work at Loyola, Ozar is also in his twenty-third year as a member of the Institutional Ethics Committee, Evanston Northwestern Healthcare, Evanston, Illinois. He was a member of the Research Review Committee of the Chicago Department of Health (1986–1993), was consulting ethicist for the Midwest Hospice and Palliative Care Center (1989–1998), and is currently a member of the Ethics Board of the Illinois Department of Children and Family Services. He has published two books and more than a hundred professional articles and book chapters on ethical issues in health care, in the professions, and in other institutions, organizations, and social systems, as well as on goals and strategies for ethics education for college, university, and professional learners.

Toby L. Schonfeld, PhD, is associate professor of healthcare ethics in the Section on Humanities and Law, Department of Preventive and Societal Medicine, at the University of Nebraska Medical Center (UNMC). She received her MA and PhD in philosophy with a concentration in medical ethics from the University of Tennessee, Knoxville. She has been at UNMC since August 2001. Dr. Schonfeld teaches in the integrated clinical experience curriculum for first- and second-year medical students and codirects the fourth-year elective on spirituality and health care. She also teaches healthcare ethics to students in the School of Allied Health Professions. She has developed Web courses in healthcare ethics and in critical thinking. Dr. Schonfeld serves on a number of committees and in several national organizations. She is vice chair of the Medical Ethics Committee and serves on the Ethics Consultation Service. She also serves on the IRB and chaired the Contraception Subcommittee. She is the secretary/treasurer of the national Society of Jewish Ethics, the editor-in-chief of the *Newsletter of the International Network on Feminist Approaches to Bioethics,* and the coordinator of the Philosophy Affinity Group for the American Society of Bioethics and Humanities. Her research interests fall into four categories: women's issues, research ethics, Jewish bioethics, and ethics education.

Wayne Shelton, PhD, MSW, earned his doctorate in philosophy from the University of Tennessee, with a concentration in medical ethics. He also has a master's in social work from the University of Chicago with a certificate in health administration and policy from the Harris School of Public Policy, and he was a fellow at the McClean Center for Medical Ethics, University of Chicago Medical Center. He is currently associate professor and director of the Program on Ethics and Health Outcomes in the Alden March Bioethics Institute at the Albany Medical Center and codirector of the AMC/Union graduate program in bioethics. Dr. Shelton's research activity has focused on ethical issues in the physician-patient relationship, medical futility, and the challenges of ethics education in medical schools. He has published in professional journals, has coedited three books, and is coeditor of the book series "Advances in Bioethics." Most recently, he is currently principal investigator of a study in the intensive care unit to measure the impact of multidisciplinary model of family support, including ethics consultation, on family satisfaction and length of stay.

Alissa Hurwitz Swota, PhD, is an assistant professor of philosophy at the University of North Florida and senior fellow in bioethics at the Blue Cross Blue Shield of Florida Center for Ethics, Public Policy, and the Professions. She completed a postdoctoral fellowship in clinical ethics at the University of Toronto Joint Centre for Bioethics. Her areas of interest include ethical issues at the end of life, clinical ethics, and cultural issues in the clinical setting.